101 Fitness Myths
Turbocharge Your Workouts to Get Leaner and Stronger Faster

Maik Wiedenbach, CPT (NASM)

CONTENTS

Part IV Supplements   105

Part V Lifestyle   120

94. My job does not allow me to make gains
95. Bodybuilding requires me to be socially awkward, which
    means I can't do it
96. I am too old to get in shape
97. Vegetarians cannot build muscle
98. Organic food is better for you
99. I can drink alcohol and still build muscle and burn fat
100.   I have a slow metabolism; that's why I am overweight
101.   I travel a lot, which makes it impossible to eat healthy

Introduction

This is the book I wish I'd had when I began weight training 20 years ago. It would have saved me so much time and frustration. That's what I want to do for you now. This book is for novices—whether you're new to the gym or have been working out religiously for years and are frustrated because you don't see the results you wish for. And to clarify, by novice I mean anyone who cannot bench press their body weight for 10 to 12 reps and dead lift twice their body weight (women should figure two-thirds of these guidelines). So if you're not there or don't even know what a dead lift is, you're a novice.

And that's a great place to be because if you're willing to put in the effort, you have the potential to achieve dramatic results in 8 to 10 weeks. I'm not talking about achieving the physique of a professional bodybuilder but a beach body you can be proud of; and that's something anyone can (and should) achieve.

When people go to the gym regularly and don't see results, they naturally get frustrated. This leads to three possible outcomes: they end up quitting the gym, abusing steroids (which, in many cases still doesn't deliver results), or developing unhealthy eating habits aka fad and crash diets.

It is my hope that this book will help you find a different way. If you can dedicate 45 minutes 3 x a week to a lifting program and maintain a reasonable diet as outlined in the following chapters, you will see great results. This book is based on a no-nonsense natural training approach to lifting weights that will get you in shape in the shortest possible time. I don't believe in wasting time at the gym. If you keep your goal in mind—whether it be losing weight, looking better, improving sports performance, or recovering from injury—you may well find that you're spending less time at the gym and seeing results like you never have before.

WORKING OUT VERSUS TRAINING

Training is different from working out. Working out is merely showing up at the gym and going through the motions for an hour or so. If you want to achieve your goals, working out is not enough. You need to commit yourself to training. Most people approach training like homework, a piece of paper that says 3x10 bench press (3 sets, 10 reps of bench press). But it's more than that; you need to feel your muscles working, feel the rep speed, and above all push yourself. Some days you add sets, some days you drop some. It's not about going through the motions; it's about improving every week.

Training requires a goal, and your training must be oriented toward achieving that goal. As a results-oriented personal trainer, I work with my clients to establish their goals before we do anything. If you don't know where you're going, there's no way you're going to get there. And goals must be specific. People often say they have a goal, but they don't really. For instance getting in shape is not a goal; it's too vague. You have to be specific. Do you want to lose 8 pounds? Be able to bench press another 20 pounds? Become a better tennis player? Improve an injured knee or shoulder? Getting in shape means nothing until you establish what it means for you specifically.

And once you have a goal, you need a plan. Whether it's a 6-week or 3-month plan, you need to evaluate your progress. Ask yourself: Where am I? Am I on track? If not, what is wrong? Maybe I'm not getting enough sleep or enough protein or maybe I'm not pushing myself hard enough in the gym.

Whatever is standing in the way of your progress can only be adjusted for if you're clear in regards to your goal and you're taking the time to evaluate your progress. And yes, sometimes life happens. You're having a stressful time on the job, you're in the midst of a divorce, you have young children keeping you up at night, you're traveling a lot—all of these can affect gym performance. Don't give up, just acknowledge the issue and find ways to correct for it.

NATURAL TRAINING

When I started training in the early 1990s, the problem was not enough information. Today with glossy fitness magazines and the Internet, we are overloaded with information. And as we're bombarded with truths, half-truths, and outright fallacies, it's easy to lose track of the basics, which is really all you need. The rest is hype, gimmicks, and marketing.

This book attempts to sift through some these myths and gimmicks in a scientific and rational manner. Most fitness books provide very little content and are mostly filled with pictures and recipes. This book is intended to make you a smarter "gym rat," making you self-sufficient in creating your routine and diet as opposed to being a slave to a trainer or the latest "breakthroughs" in the magazines.

Aside from the experience that I have gained through my years as a professional athlete and trainer of an exclusive clientele in Manhattan, I believe strongly in keeping up to date with the latest scientific research on training, fitness, and nutrition. For those who are interested in the research that informed the conclusions in this book, I have provided a suggested reading list.

As a natural trainee, especially if you have family, a job, and a life, you have to take into account that you only have limited recoverability. So you'll need to customize your workouts to be brief, to the point, and efficient. The novice natural trainee should focus on 2 to 3 45-minute whole body workouts per week. And to make the most efficient use of your time, emphasize multi-muscle exercises. The squat hits 200 muscles at once, whereas an abdominal crunch hits 3. What's more effective if you have limited time? The answer is that most novices will see much quicker progress with 2 to 3 whole body workouts a week than following the latest 6-day split routine.

Although this is a book for natural trainees, I deal with steroids in a very straightforward way here for two reasons. First, steroid use is behind many of the myths that hold back the natural trainee. Second, no matter what warnings I might give—and make no mistake, steroid use is a felony in the U.S. and if you get caught, you are in serious trouble—steroid use is extremely common in the bodybuilding world.

Because I have written this book for the natural trainee, I am mainly concerned here with how the proliferation of steroids is a source of major frustration for the novice. Do not fall into the trap of comparing your physique and your progress to steroid-enhanced bodies—it's like comparing apples and oranges. Steroids work; they work extremely well in aiding muscle recovery. They provide testosterone and improve glycogen storage, and because they allow muscles to recover faster, a person taking steroids can train longer and harder. The natural trainee is in a completely different world, meaning if you train like them, you are going to lose your muscle by over training and ultimately burn out.

As a natural trainee without the artificial muscle protection of steroids, you must pay as much attention to recovery time between workouts as you do to your routine in the gym. Training is a lifestyle; the real work begins outside the gym where eating healthy foods and getting enough rest are going to be your challenges.

Lifting routines targeting specific muscles are a staple of the glossy fitness magazines. They usually print the routine of some guy (or often make up a routine) who won a title, but most of these guys are on 25 different pharmaceuticals; so whatever applies to him has nothing to do with the natural trainee. As a novice you don't need a 20-set bicep program. Besides the near certainty that he takes steroids, he has been working out for 20 plus years. He's at a different level than you, and you and he have nothing in common. So, anything you read from these people, take it with a grain of salt. Be wary of gimmicky approaches, such as split training (exercising only one body part on different days), which originated with the advent of steroids.

For the natural trainee with a life, it's just not feasible. You would need to devote hours to training every day; you'd have to move to the gym. It's not practical. Most people who are not taking steroids and who try split training get injured, burned out, or just frustrated, and they conclude that they just can't get in shape because they're not gifted. In reality, they are just overtraining and undereating.

ANYONE CAN BE IN SHAPE

Weightlifting works for anybody—men, women, old, young, lean, or large—because it's logical. Anybody can make progress, great progress. Anybody can get results because it's a natural progression: you challenge your body, feed it properly, and it will respond. Your body will make thicker muscle fibers, and it will get leaner.

And yes, there are genetic differences among people, but everyone has the potential for an amazing physique. People are different, so it follows that certain exercises are better for certain people. For instance, some people might not be made for squatting, but they can do dumbbell squats, or siff lunges; there's a whole realm of things they can do. And different people will progress at different rates. Some people might change dramatically in 3 months while others might take 9 months.

People over 55 do have a harder time building muscle because of reduced testosterone levels, but you can still build muscle at any age if you're diligent with your diet. You can't train as often as younger people and you can't train as heavy. But by training you will elevate your testosterone levels and growth hormone levels and increase body stability. That's particularly significant for women because weight training can help prevent osteoporosis.

Images of young beautiful lean muscular men and women abound today in fitness magazines, television advertisements, billboards—seemingly everywhere you turn. One of the very unfortunate side effects of these images is that average mortals have been led to believe that these few blessed people are the only ones who can get in shape. Average mortals internalize this as an excuse for not getting in shape: "I'm just not one of the gifted people, it's not my fault, and I'm powerless to change." This could not be further from the truth. Everyone's muscles are the same and respond to weight training and diet. Anyone can have 6-pack abs—the key is to reduce your body fat percentage so that the muscles are visible.

EVERY BODY IS DIFFERENT

In physique building if you're mindful of your food, your sleep, and your training, you will look good. The question is how long will it take you. Some people get there quicker, others slower. But you must take responsibility for your own development.

And if you were in shape at an earlier time in your life and have fallen off the wagon, take heart. Muscle has memory, believe it or not. So somebody who has been in shape, no matter how long ago will get back in shape quicker than someone who was never in shape.

I work with a lot of women in my training practice and I always tell them if you look at men's and women's muscle cells under a microscope, there's no difference. The differences are in the testosterone levels, distribution of muscle fibers, joints, and stability. In general, women can't lift as heavy as men. But although they can't train in the 100% zone as well as men, women have greater endurance so that they can lift in the 85% range for longer than men. Women in training often have different goals and areas of focus. While men most often concentrate on upper body, women's goals tend towards the lower body where they have more muscle fibers but also tend to accumulate more fat.

So, while there are some differences as to how to approach training, women should absolutely lift weights. Weight training will do more for a woman's health than cardio alone ever could. For women there's no better butt lift, so to speak, than deadlifts. It is more efficient than any treadmill or elliptical at shaping up your butt. And studies have shown that weight training can be of great benefit in warding off osteoporosis.

And no, women do not get big from weight training. Women have about 1/16 of the testosterone of men. If you think how hard it is for the average guy to gain muscle and you divide that by 16, you have a woman. So women do not have to worry about growing that much muscle. Also, muscle has only 35%the mass of body fat; so if you build 2 pounds of muscle and you lose 2 pounds of fat, you will be smaller than you were before even though you weigh the same.

DIET IS 80% OF YOUR APPEARANCE

Your diet is 80% of what you look like. You can work out like a maniac, but if your diet is off, it will never lead to anything. In fact if one person works out and has a crappy diet, and the other has a good diet and doesn't work out, the one who doesn't work out will look better. You cannot out-exercise poor diet, no matter how hard you try.

On the flip side you cannot pump up your appearance on a strict diet without exercising. The body is an ingenious machine, programmed for survival. If you starve your body, it will treat muscle as a luxury. Since muscle maintenance costs are much higher than those of fat deposits. It is "use it or lose it." During a strict diet, when fuel (food) is scarce, fat deposits are valuable and the muscles burn all the resources. So, they are reduced to the size necessary to perform the tasks of an "effort-free" lifestyle and reduce energy consumption. Fat will remain until all other expendable energy sources are depleted.

Once the diet ends, pounds will be gone, but very little of the weight lost is actually body fat. You will end up losing mostly muscle. You've set yourself up for an undesirable low muscle to fat ratio, causing the metabolic rate to plummet, setting off the dreaded "Yo-Yo" effect (the rapid regain of the same or higher number of pounds as you had lost).

AEROBIC EXERCISE IS NOT ENOUGH

While cardio training does have benefits, it is the slowest way to burn body fat because it lowers your metabolic rate. When doing cardio, the body burns muscles and fat indifferently, so while you lose size, your body fat percentage does not change that much. Cardio does not build muscle; so it cannot alter your body composition—increasing your muscle to fat ratio, is the most effective way to increase your metabolic rate.

Every day in the gym I see men and women pedaling away for hours on elliptical trainers, Stairmasters, and stationary bicycles, and it's not getting them the body they're after. The truth is that cardio basically makes you better at cardio. Cardio does expend energy and burn calories, but the problem is your body is very good at adjusting to that. The more cardio you do, the more efficient your body gets so that you have to do that much more just to stay even. It's a game of diminishing returns and not a very efficient use of training time.

The other problem with cardio is that the calories you expend are not necessarily from your fat stores. You have no control over where your body pulls the calories. They can be from your glycogen stores, fat cells, or muscle protein. This is why runners have no upper body mass—all the arms, shoulders, chest, and back muscles get cannibalized to produce the energy needed.

THE TWO BEST SUPPLEMENTS YOU CAN BUY

If you're serious about training, you should have two logbooks: one for your food, and one for your lifting. These logbooks are the two best supplements you'll ever buy. And they're also cheap. Buy a little notebook, write on a piece of paper, type into your phone—whatever works for you. Because if you find you're not progressing, the answer is always there in the logbooks. Maybe you have been eating too much, or eating too little, or maybe you're stuck on an exercise that's not working for you—in order to progress you have to know what to change. On that last point, people do tend to get into a comfort zone; they like to do certain exercises, other's not so much. They keep doing the ones they like and ignore the others. The logbook will point the way out of your rut.

IMPROVING YOUR BODY BOOSTS YOUR CONFIDENCE

One of the most remarkable benefits of bodybuilding is not the physical reward but how success in shaping your body can improve your outlook on life. Taking control of and shaping your body gives you a tremendous boost in self-confidence and wellbeing, and that feeling of success spills over into other areas of your life. I can tell you from experience that the sense of empowerment you gain from training can be a tremendous help in tumultuous times. So often, life comes at us like a tsunami and it's all we can do to keep our heads above water. In the gym, on the other hand, there's nothing that you can't control. Lifting 100 pounds will always be lifting 100 pounds. You have your goal, you have your workout, and it gives you a sense of order.

I'm giving pro bono training to an underprivileged kid right now. He does not have an easy life, but it's tremendously gratifying to see the boost in confidence he gets from training and seeing the results. The effect is similar with clients, who've gone through a divorce and put on weight and then come to me. The sense of control in one area of their lives spills over into other areas of their lives.

This book is for people who want to improve their bodies but who cannot dedicate a large amount of time to physical training because they have a life. You can achieve a better physique than you ever thought possible if you can do 2 to 3 whole body workouts a week; eat sensibly, simply, and low carb (unless you are one of the lucky ones who can handle carbs well); track and evaluate your food and exercise progress, and have a positive mind set. Keep challenging your muscles and your mind!

Part I
Weight Training

1. I don't have the genetics
2. A pro routine will make me big
3. Pros have secret exercises
4. I am a hard gainer
5. Dead lifts are bad for your lower back
6. Squats are bad for your knees
7. Flat bench is the best exercise for chest
8. I want to transform my fat into muscle
9. Shaping versus bulking exercise: What's the difference?
10. You need to do barbell curls for your biceps
11. Women need different exercises than men
12. Women need to lift lower weights and higher repetitions than men
13. No pain no gain
14. Aspirin helps with soreness
15. I don't train legs because I already ride my bike, play soccer, etc.
16. More sets are better
17. A split program is the best way to work out
18. High intensity training (HIT) is the best way to gain mass
19. I want to look like…
20. A wide grip works the outer parts of the muscle
21. Squats give you a big butt
22. You can alter the shape of your muscles by performing certain exercises
23. Women should not lift weights because it will make them bulky
24. Low repetitions are for bulking
25. You need a pump for muscles to grow
26. You need to go to failure on every set during every workout
27. Ab blaster, ab roller, ab wheel, the super ab machine
28. Electro stimulation helps to grow muscle
29. Bodybuilders aren't really strong
30. You need to stretch before lifting weights
31. Weightlifting stunts growth therefore kids shouldn't lift weights
32. Isometrics build muscle
33. You can reduce body fat in a spot

34. Go heavy or go home
35. Once you stop training all the muscle will turn to fat
36. You have to eat big to get big
37. Free weights are better than machines
38. Ab- and adductor machines are great for slimming thighs
39. Weight training makes you stiff and inflexible
40. Cheat repetitions are good for muscle growth

1.   I don't have the genetics

I hear this a lot—both in the gym and casual conversation. Genetics are a favorite scapegoat for athletic shortcomings. We blame genetics for our failure to build muscle or lose body fat. But how much do genetics really influence your success in the gym? The answer is less than you would like to believe. While everyone has inherited a certain blueprint, which includes having good and not-so-good muscle groups, certain hormonal levels, and fat storage tendencies, it is also true that ANYONE can get in amazing shape. You are trying to build the best body for you, not to emulate someone else.

Think of your body as a plant. Given the right conditions, a plant will grow and blossom. If it doesn't, that means something is wrong— a parasite, not enough light, or too much water, perhaps. The same applies to your body: There is always an explanation for why you're not progressing. Success in training has 3 pillars: training, recovery, and nutrition. Most people at best get 2 out of 3 right.

Most of us don't have the potential of Arnold Schwarzenegger, but that doesn't mean we cannot achieve our own goals. By way of example, look at a guy competing against Arnold: Frank Zane. He had narrow clavicles, a long torso, 16-inch arms, and weighed 190 pounds at a height of 5'10". In short, he had one of the worst possible genetic make-ups for a pro bodybuilder. Yet, he won Mr. Olympia 3 times, beating Arnold!

How did he do it? He stuck to his diet, trained with unmatched intensity, and did not take no for an answer. He realized that he couldn't compete with Arnold on the basis of mass; so he created the most symmetrical physique, which many people still consider as close to perfect as a human can get.

Frank Zane's story is inspiring. Your first step is to honestly assess yourself, your schedule, and your training experience, and devise the plan that's right for you. What is my goal? Mass in the upper body? Lean legs?

If your progress has been snail-like, then you might need to work out less often to give your body enough recovery time. Another approach would be to focus on certain body parts that you deem weaker and train them twice a week. Look at your body like a piece of art. You are the artist; it's up to you to create the perfect physique for your particular body. For example, if you have wide hips, don't waste your time with oblique training to make your hips narrow; train your shoulders instead. The wider your shoulders are, the narrower your waist will appear.

Also, stop working out and start training. Training means, "to increase the capacity to perform a skill or work." If you are still training with the same weights after 12 months, you are simply not better. Push yourself to the limit in every workout to achieve your goals. Training is a lifestyle; whereas working out is neat and cute like a French class you take every 2 weeks. The only way you'll really learn French is by moving to France and speaking only French.

The same applies to your body; it is a 24/7 project—training, eating, resting, and learning.

Remember, creating a physique is not a race against other people. You are doing this for yourself. If someone else gets in shape quicker or with seemingly less effort, don't be discouraged. Don't psych yourself out with complaints about your genetics because you can't change them. The time you spend complaining could be much better used cooking a healthy meal or working out.

2.   A pro routine will make me big

A routine that supposedly got Mr. Olympia to where he is will most likely not work for you. By the same token, asking the biggest guy for advice is probably the worst mistake you can make during your quest for a better body.

Here's why: Pro bodybuilders can train at a much higher level since they hold several advantages over you: superior genetics, the ability to sleep 8 hours a night, and eating 6 to 7 meals a day. If you look at pictures of top athletes as young people, they are already more muscular and leaner than their counterparts. They tend to store less body fat and push nutrients into the muscle, which is why they can consume 5,000 calories a day without becoming obese.

And yes, there are drugs, a whole plethora of them, which enable them to diet more strictly and recover more quickly. There are anabolic steroids, growth hormone, insulin, diet drugs, thyroid medication, appetite suppressants, fat burners, and plenty more.

Anyone who tells you that this type of development can be achieved without drugs is lying or trying to sell you a supplement.

The average person, who has to deal with job, family, and career, simply cannot maintain such a demanding regime. If you're like most of us, you just have to carefully track your progress and adjust your routine accordingly. Ask yourself every 10 weeks: Am I getting stronger? Can I do more repetitions? Am I leaner? If after several months the answer to all these questions is no, you need to adjust your routine and diet. Overtraining could be one of the problems.

If you haven't progressed in the gym for several weeks, take a week or 10 days off from the gym. You can take up other sports for a while, but rest as much as possible. While you're resting, keep your calories slightly elevated without eating a lot of junk food. Many trainees are over-trained and underfed; so the combination of rest and food can produce amazing gains.

While your body is given a chance to recover and rebuild, you should use that time to come up with a new personal routine for the next 8 to 10 weeks and then stick to it. When the 8 to 10 weeks are up, it's time to reevaluate (pictures or an honest friend can be very helpful) and plan your next step.

3.   Pros have secret exercises

If you observe a pro or world-class athlete training, whether on DVD or in real life, you will realize that their routines do not reinvent the wheel. Most workouts are very basic and revolve around the meat-and-potato exercises such as the squat and bench press. So how are they able to achieve more dramatic results than the rest of us?

To begin with, these athletes tend to have a bone structure more favorable to packing on muscle (broad shoulders with a small waist). What's more, they tend to be naturally lean and are able to process nutrients much more efficiently. They also know intuitively when to rest, i.e., they are less likely to over-train. Overtraining is one of the biggest pitfalls for most people since they don't eat or rest enough to achieve maximum results. If you haven't progressed during the last 8 to 10 months despite putting sufficient effort into the gym, a week off with a slightly higher caloric intake might just be the cure.

Most importantly, though, what separates world-class athletes from the average trainees is an amazing mind-muscle connection. These individuals are able to fully focus on the particular muscle they are working and, in so doing, achieve much higher muscle-fiber activation per set. This makes their training sessions significantly more productive. So it is not the exercise itself but how the exercise is performed that separates world-class athletes from the rest of us.

The next time you are at the gym, leave your ego at the door and visualize the muscle you are attempting to train. Studying an anatomy chart and learning how muscles move and where they are located can also help. When starting your workout, it would be wise to spend one set doing the motion very slowly, with light weight, and focus on squeezing and releasing your target muscle. Don't just move weights; try to engage your target muscles on every rep and every set.

This will enable you to train with greater efficiency during the remainder of the workout. Little improvements will lead to big gains!

4.   I am a hard gainer

Hard gainer might be one of the most overused terms in bodybuilding and is frequently confused with the somatype of an ectomorph. When most people refer to a hard gainer, they mean someone who has a harder time putting on muscle mass than other people. So called hard gainers often experience frustration and disillusion and turn to steroid use in order to make up for their perceived handicap.

But what really is a hard gainer and, more importantly, is he or she a hopeless case? Typically, a hard gainer has long limbs, narrow clavicles, and a tendency to be very lean. So is this person doomed in the quest for an amazing physique?

Not at all. In truth, the hard gainer's natural leanness is a big advantage. A leaner physique always looks better when it's developed than a body that is 20 pounds heavier and whose muscular development is obscured by water and fat. A hard gainer only needs to put on 5 to 10 pounds of muscle mass in order to achieve a dramatic visual change.

You don't need to weigh 240 pounds in order to appear muscular when 5 pounds of lean mass on the shoulders and upper chest is probably enough to go from scrawny to brawny.

There are, however, some things a hard gainer should bear in mind. First, since most hard gainers have limited recovery ability, sessions should be kept brief and intense. Forty-five minutes at the most and no more than 16 to 18 sets total for the entire workout. Second, train only 3 times a week, focusing on basic exercises and making sure you get a pump. Third, get 8 hours of sleep. If you can take a nap in the afternoon, even better. Try to avoid all stimulants, such as caffeine, since they can impair your recovery.

Fourth, a hard gainer needs to eat at least 500 calories over maintenance (bodyweight in pounds multiplied by 16 for most trainees) in order to build quality muscle mass. Stick to mainly clean foods in a 35% protein/40% carbohydrates/25% fat ratio, distributed over 5 to 6 meals a day. An athlete with 200 pounds bodyweight would need 3,700 calories, 600 calories per meal and 5 to 6 meals a day. Four of those meals should be solid, plus the pre- and post-workout shakes; make sure to keep it a clean bulk. You want to gain quality muscle mass, not just weight.

In my experience, people that claim to be hard gainers are often terrified of getting fat and therefore do not take in sufficient calories. Some coaches even go as far as to say: There are no hard gainers, just under eaters. Keep in mind, Frank Zane was the quintessential hard gainer, and he built one of the best physiques ever!

5.   Dead lifts are bad for your lower back

Actually, the opposite is true. Dead lifts, if done properly, are probably the single best exercise to develop strength and mass in the erector spinae. These muscles are crucial to lower back health since they hold the spine firmly between them. The stronger and more stable these muscles are, the more support they will give to your lower back. Considering that two-thirds of Americans suffer from back pain at some point in their lives, deadlifts should be a staple of anyone who exercises.

What's more, the dead lift incorporates a wide array of muscles, such as trapezius, abdominals, calves, quadriceps, and hamstrings that makes it an excellent choice for developing the overall body. It is also an anabolic accelerator for body recomposition (gaining muscle and losing fat) because it triggers the release of growth hormone and testosterone, which are two of the most powerful muscle-conditioning hormones in the body.

If you do not have a pre-existing back condition that prohibits you from doing this exercise, you should definitely add it to your workout. The two most crucial technique points are to look forward, never downward and to keep the bar close to your legs at all times. This will prevent you from rounding your back during the movement. By doing dead lifts, you are putting your body into a more anabolic state, which will help you achieve your goals quicker. So don't shy away from them, use them to your advantage.

6.   Squats are bad for your knees

Most people who say this are simply not willing to squat because it is a very demanding exercise. As for knee injuries, the leg extension does much more harm to the knee because it is open ended, placing undue stress on the patella. The squat, on the other hand, is a grounded exercise. The squat is a very functional and natural movement that follows the way your knee was intended to move. All major leg muscles (quadriceps, hamstrings and gluteus) have to work together in this exercise in order to lift the weight. In order to get the most out of a squat, choose a weight that allows you to squat with good form all the way down and up. Again, it's all about technique. With the toes pointed out (imagine standing on a clock, one foot pointed at 1 pm, the other one at 11 am) and a proper positioning of the upper body (push your chest out, keep your gaze upward), the stress on the knees is greatly reduced. One of the common mistakes is to use too much weight and only perform half squats thereby creating a shearing force on the bones in the knee.

Another very typical mistake is to lean too far forward at the low point of the exercise. This is usually caused by a weak lower back which should be strengthened with hyperextensions and dead lifts.

Although there is some compression of the knee joint at the low point of the squat, the forces on the knee ligaments are moderate and comfortably in the tolerance range. The knee joint is flexing and extending concurrently with the hip and ankle, which means the muscles learn to produce force in an integrated fashion. The exercise is also ground-based which makes it a much safer choice over leg extensions and leg curls. To perform it correctly, the athlete must retain balance and alignment of the knee and stability of the lower back during the entire motion. All these factors mean that for either rehabilitating the knee joint and/or developing strength in the quadriceps, the squat is a high-value exercise.

In addition, like the dead lift, the squat causes a release of serum testosterone, which leads to greater overall gains.

Famous iron guru Vince Gironda used to have his trainees start even their arm workouts with hack squats because he believed that the hormonal optimization would yield bigger biceps!

7. Flat bench is the best exercise for chest

Tell someone in the continental US that you work out and you will invariably be asked, '"what do you bench?" People seem to consider the bench one of the most important exercises, especially the male population (bragging rights included). But is it really the best thing you can do for your chest? That depends on a number of variables such as arm length, muscle awareness, size of your rib cage, shoulder versus triceps development, and other factors. While the flat bench is without a doubt a useful tool in developing a big chest, there are also other exercises, which are just as beneficial, such as the incline press, dips, and the dumbbell bench press. One trainee might get great results from the flat bench while his friend will only develop tendonitis in the shoulder. It is important to keep an open mind and not to be too dogmatic. In the end you need to feel the muscle working, not your joints creaking. Many bodybuilders swear by dips and or dumbbell presses for their chest development and achieve great results.

I personally believe that the flat bench creates unnecessary stress on your shoulders and that there are better ways to build your pectorals. There, I said it: I don't like the flat bench as a pectoral builder. Most people tend to use too much weight and bounce the bar of their chest without properly activating their target muscles. Bodybuilding is about developing a physique not just moving weights from point A to point B.

A new way to look at an old classic

Vince Gironda did not have any flat benches in his gym because he felt they created a "droopy" chest. His favorite exercise was the weighted dip, which produced great results in many of his trainees. One has to remember that the primary function of the pectorals is to move the arm laterally across the body; therefore the incorporation of a fly or cross over movement in your chest training is a must.

Sometimes even a different grip or angle can work wonders. I would also try different numbers of repetitions and varying the speeds at which you do the exercise. For some weeks you could train with an 8x8 system, then switch to a traditional power pyramid, such as 12, 10, 8, and then 6 repetitions. After 6 weeks of that, I would try an integrated power/stretch/pump approach.

If your chest is lagging, try to train it twice a week and use visualization techniques, such as squeezes and side chest poses in front of the mirror in order to connect with your muscle.
Don't be afraid to try new things, but also don't be haphazard and switch every week. You need to give each approach enough time to tell whether it's working for you.

I would give any combination of exercises and rep numbers 6 weeks to prove themselves. If after 6 weeks no change has occurred (provided you did not change your diet), it is time to try something new.

8.   I want to transform my fat into muscle

Trying to transform fat into muscle is like trying to turn lead into gold as alchemists tried unsuccessfully to do throughout the Middle Ages. Muscle and fat have two entirely different chemical structures and one cannot be transformed into the other. You can only increase your muscle mass and decrease the fat content of your body. But here's the trick: both goals require mutually exclusive starting points so they can't be pursued at the same time.

Building muscle is a hypercaloric process, meaning you will have to eat above maintenance whereas losing fat requires a calorie deficit. Building muscle and losing weight are diametrically opposed with regard to their nutritional requirements as well as the hormonal state they require the body to be in. It is advisable to plan the year in 10 or 12 week cycles. Give yourself 2 to 3 months to gain muscle and then diet for 8 weeks.

Building muscle and losing fat

The main obstacle any trainee faces when trying to reshape the body is nutrition partitioning. In a perfect universe every calorie you ate would go into the muscle tissue, so you would be 100% muscle. Conversely, any calorie you didn't eat while dieting would be pulled from fat storage so you would never lose any muscle.

Unfortunately, the universe is not perfect. When building muscle you always gain some fat; when dieting, you always lose some muscle.

While you can minimize these effects through a nutrient rotation and intelligent training, you can't totally avoid them. Training and eating can influence about 30% of this process. The rest is genetics (your hormonal levels of testosterone and T-3), which will decide how much fat you gain or muscle you lose. This does not apply for steroid users since they create an artificially perfect hormonal environment.

So as a natural trainee, you will have to accept that for every 2 to 3 pounds of muscle that you build, you will also gain up to 1 pound of fat. Monitor the fat gain very closely, since it is very hard to get rid of new fat cells. For a long time it was believed that adults couldn't build new fat cells, however it seems that this is exactly what happens. Unfortunately, it seems that we cannot build new muscle cells. Life is unfair.

During the diet you will lose up to 1 pound of muscle along with every 2 to 3 pounds of fat lost. So the balance in the universe is restored. Most people who try to gain muscle and lose fat at the same time usually end up failing at both. Only rank beginners or steroid users can get away with achieving both but even then, only for a very short period of time. Therefore, you must set yourself a time frame and keep in mind that every week you can either lose 2 pounds of fat or gain half a pound of muscle. Before embarking on this journey, you will need to determine how much fat you want to lose (or muscle to gain) and design your diet and workout accordingly.

Creating a physique does not happen in a straight line. You should think of it as three steps forward, one step back. It is a marathon, not a sprint.

9. Shaping versus bulking exercises: What's the difference?

One of the most misunderstood topics in bodybuilding is the belief that there are some exercises that shape or define the muscle and others that bulk it up. Unfortunately, the shape or form of a muscle is genetically predetermined and cannot be altered.

Just to give you an example, the incline bench is usually seen as a bulk exercise for the chest, while cable flyes are seen as a shaping exercise. While performing either exercise, however, the pectorals simply contract and relax. So where does th s notion come from?

Most likely, it occurs that heavy benching is done in the off-season, when people are stronger and bigger. During a diet, especially when an athlete is eating fewer carbohydrates and therefore has less energy, many athletes don't have the strength to perform heavy bench anymore so they resort to cable flyes for a chest workout. Since they are leaner, they conclude that the cable flyes must have done the trick, not the dramatically reduced calories and increased cardio.

So are all exercises created equal? Not quite. In my opinion, when training a muscle it is necessary to perform a mid range or power movement and follow that up with a stretch exercise.

As an example, for the chest, one would do incline presses followed by dumbbell flyes with an emphasis on the stretch. The big exercise involves a lot of other muscles such as the triceps and the shoulders and forces the body to release growth hormone during the workout. Following with a stretch motion, the athlete creates tissue tears, which will enable further muscle growth. The body needs to repair those tears, which consumes a lot of energy (fat loss) and makes the muscle stronger (muscle gain) depending on your caloric intake.

This could be finished with a pump set of push-ups in order to maximize blood flow into the muscle. Better blood flow means more nutrients and oxygen, the perfect set up for progress. This program can be found in the book *Critical Mass: The Positions of Flexion Approach to Explosive Muscle Growth,* by Steve Holman. It is an excellent work, I highly recommend it.

10. You need to do barbell curls for your biceps

Before I start I want to make one thing clear: Never be a slave to a routine, even if you wrote it. If you don't get a mind-muscle connection with the muscle during that exercise or workout, move on and find something else. In general, people are too concerned with their 3x10 routine, treating it as if it were homework. Training is about improving your capacity to work, not to do three sets of X.

With that said, what is the deal with barbell curls? Just like with barbell bench presses, the effects you will get from barbell curls very much depends on your body type. Anyone who has ever seen *Pumping Iron* with Arnold working his arms won't doubt the effectiveness of this particular exercise, but there are other valid options such as cable curls, EZ bar (bent barbell), and dumbbells. People with long forearms will have a harder time with the barbell curl and might be prone to inflammation of the wrist (as I am). The EZ bar would be a better choice for those people.

Not all arms are created equal. Often the stronger arm will take over during a barbell curl, diminishing the workload of the weaker one. The dumbbell curl would be a good way to find out which arm is weaker. In addition, you could then perform 1 to 2 extra sets just on the weaker side in order to establish equilibrium. Even Arnold had about a 1 inch size difference between his left and right biceps.

The brachioradialis muscle runs under your biceps' brachii and pushes them up, giving them the much-desired peak. To work out this muscle, do reverse curls and the long-forgotten Zottman curl. Another good investment would be to by a pair of Fatgripz and use them on dumbbell and barbell exercises. They will force you to work your forearms harder, and will contribute to overall arm growth.

Studies have also shown that the close grip pull up causes the greatest activation in the muscle fibers of the biceps. So, try the pull up bar for bigger biceps!

11. Women need different exercises than men

Despite what a certain popular relationship book says, men and women are from the same planet.

The female body has the same structure as male body with the same muscles, joints, and ligaments. The main difference lies in the hormonal make up. Men have more testosterone than women, which means they can be stronger, leaner, and have more stable joints. Hormones don't influence the selection of exercises a man or woman should do, only the amount of weight they should lift. And, while women can't lift as heavy (due to their lack of testosterone and their bone structure) that doesn't mean they should not try to lift as much weight as possible!

The main reason women should lift heavy weights with intensity is because it's the fastest way to change your physique, no matter who you are. Under a microscope a female muscle cell looks exactly like a male muscle cell. This means both sexes can benefit from the same pattern of training. Muscle needs a catalyst in order to change, and for women that catalyst is training at 85% capacity. Only intense training will cause the adaptive processes in the body such as strength gain and fat loss. The only difference in training for women is with regard to weights moved. A woman's 1 repetition max (1RM) tends to be lower than a male's. This is because female muscles have a lower activation of fibers, meaning their neuromuscular efficiency is not as high as men's. Their strength output is lower. They may not be able to lift as heavy, but interestingly, women are able to perform for a longer period of time at a 90% level. That needs to be taken into account when designing a training program.

So, while there is no such thing as training for women versus training for men, women tend to have different areas of focus. Whereas men like to work on chest and arms, women tend to be more concerned with their lower body, legs, and gluteus. Man or woman, you should always construct your program to meet your personal goals and work your weakest points first.

As an example for weak point training, women tend to be quad dominant, meaning their hamstrings are much weaker than their quadriceps, which can lead to knee injuries. So women might want to include plenty of hamstring raises, stiff legged dead lifts, and leg curls in their workouts. If you suffer from computer posture (forward slumped, with tight pectorals and deltoids), your back is too weak. You will need to prioritize rows, pull downs, and pullovers.

It is worth noting that the North American female tends to be deficient in iron and calcium, which affects performance negatively. Adding iron and calcium rich foods, such as wheat germ, dairy, and shrimp to a diet will not only result in better performance but also enhance bone stability, which is a subject of great concern to many women. Heavy lifting has also shown to be an excellent precaution against osteoporosis.

So, instead of getting hung up on training for men versus woman, keep in mind that only you know what you want your body to look like, what your weaker muscles are, if you have had any injuries and how often you can workout.

With these things in mind, design the program that's right for you.

12. Women need to lift with lower weights and higher repetitions than men

This particular myth has been around for long time and alas refuses to go away.

As previously described, the concept of toning has forced women to spend the better part of the last 30 years on the treadmill and lifting 3-pound dumbbells. However, the results, or lack thereof, speak for themselves. Most people did not achieve the lean physique they were striving for. The answer is simple: the body was not forced into a change because the resistance was not enough.

While women on average cannot lift as heavy weights as men, because they don't produce sufficient amounts of testosterone and growth hormone, they still need to train at their maximum. In order to change their bodies, women need to lift heavy and intense within their abilities.

When women talk about changing their bodies, they mostly mean losing weight—fat, to be precise. It is important to distinguish between body fat percentage and body weight: a person who is lean will look good regardless of her actual weight. The eye perceives body fat percentage, not actual body weight.

In order to lose body fat, you need to create an energy deficit. This can be achieved two ways: lower you caloric intake or increase your basic metabolic rate. I prefer and practice a combination of the two.

Here's why: sustaining muscle costs the body significantly more energy than sustaining fat. Improving your muscle to fat ratio (meaning adding more muscle, while decreasing total amount of fat) will boost your metabolism, even when resting.

Now, the most efficient way to build muscle and lose fat is by first intensely working your bigger muscles (back, chest, and legs). The larger the muscle, the more energy it will need to contract and relax. And again, remember: use increasingly heavier weights, in short sets for 6 to 10 repetitions. High repetition cycles are very time consuming and useless because they do not challenge the body enough to cause change. On the contrary, short sets with increasingly heavy weights are time efficient and keep your muscles challenged.

Simply compare the body of a marathon runner with that of a 400 meter hurdler. The hurdle sprinter is leaner and more muscular without being bulky because she is performing a short, all-out, high-intensity exercise as opposed to a 2-hour low-intensity run. The marathon runner holds more bodyfat and less muscle, due to the demands of her race. A set of heavy squats has very similar characteristics in VO2 max (the maximum capacity of someone's body to transport oxygen) and growth hormone release to the 400 meter hurdle race. You get the picture: Ladies, it's time to drop the pink dumbbells and pick up some heavy stuff!

13.   No pain no gain

Despite the example of the legendary NFL heroes playing with a broken ankle or rib, this is not a good idea._Here a distinction is necessary: muscle fatigue and soreness are fine, joint discomfort or real pain is unacceptable. Whenever this occurs, your body is sending you a pretty clear message that something is not right and you better take a break._It is then necessary to determine what causes the pain (wrong motion or muscular imbalance, for example) then take the appropriate steps to ameliorate the situation. In the case of a sprained ankle, always remember Rest, Ice, Compress and Elevate (RICE). Under no circumstances should you continue to exercise with a sprained ankle, since this might cause severe damage. Seek a qualified medical opinion._It is also not advisable to train with fever. Your body already needs all its energy to fight off the virus; it doesn't need to be further weakened by a workout. Also, you are exposing yourselves to myocarditis, an inflammatory disease of the heart, which could cause serious complications down the road.

In general, take 1 day off for every day you had a fever. Chances are you will come back stronger than you were before.

The deep soreness after a leg workout, on the other hand, should be welcomed because it indicates that you targeted the muscle properly and sent a message to change. For a long time it was assumed that muscle soreness was caused by lactic acid in the muscle. Now we know that this feeling is actually the result of microscopic tears in the muscle. In most cases even the deepest soreness will subside in 3 to 7 days. Methods to speed up healing include a warm bath or shower, gentle stretching, or getting some soft tissue work (massage of foam roll). If you performed a very heavy chest workout on Monday, it could also be a good idea to do a couple of very light sets on Wednesday to increase blood flow in the muscle.

If the soreness persists more than 7 days, you should consult a physician.

14.   Aspirin helps with soreness

First off, aspirin does help with soreness. But is it a good thing? Not really, I am afraid. Training and building muscle is an inflammatory process; the damage caused by training, triggers a bodily response. The body fights the inflammation with protein and minerals. In short, it makes the muscle stronger in order to be better equipped the next time this happens. Substances called prostaglandins (don't worry, you won't be quizzed on this) are responsible for protein synthesis in the muscle cell. Any NSAID (nonsteroidal anti-inflammatory), such as aspirin or ibuprofen, will short circuit this process and pretty much stop any growth dead in its tracks because they work as prostaglandin inhibitors. Essentially, you bust your butt in the gym for zero return!

In addition, it is not healthy to overuse these painkillers since there can be harmful interactions with the liver and stomach. A much better alternative would be fish oils, which are actually used by the body to build muscle and do not cause upset stomach. A good fish oil source would be salmon, mackerel, or fish oil capsules. A word of warning: there is such a thing as too much of a good thing. Overdosing on fish oils will lead to the same dilemma as taking NSAIDs. Stick with 6 to 9 grams daily.

Another way to combat post exercise soreness would be to consume antioxidants. Great sources here are blueberries, leafy greens, cinnamon, and grape juice. Whey protein or BCAs are extremely helpful in regards to protein synthesis and recovery. Caffeine also has some soreness relieving properties plus it works as a pre-workout stimulant and aids in fat loss.

A more mechanical option would be to perform a light workout the day after your heavy session where you would reduce your working weights by 50% and stop before muscle failure. This will cause additional blood flow into the muscle, which will speed recovery. In any event, you should consider soreness a battle scar and be proud of it!

15. I don't train legs because I already ride my bike, play soccer, etc.

Congratulations on your commitment to outdoor sports, but it will not be enough to excuse you from leg training. Did any of the past Tour de France winners strike you as someone who could win best legs at the Mr. Olympia competition?

No, because endurance sports do not build a lot of muscle. Biking is more of an aerobic activity so it doesn't give your muscles enough resistance to stimulate your legs sufficiently. It also focuses more on the quadriceps than on the hamstrings. In order to achieve sufficient leg growth, you will have to dedicate some time to the dreaded squats, lunges, and leg presses. Tennis players and skiers often have chronically underdeveloped hamstrings compared to their quadriceps despite "using their legs all the time." This can lead to knee injuries, tight IT bands (iliotibial band, which stretches from the hip to the knee on the outside of the leg) and the like. If you are a ball player, you should know that during certain moments such as landing after a basket or lunging for a long ball, the pressure on the knee could be up to 1,000 pounds. There is no better way to prepare for this than weight training.

As for the ladies, there is nothing better for a "butt lift" than lunges and stiff-legged dead lifts.

Still not convinced? Consider this: by performing squats and dead lifts you create an anabolic response in your body, which will stimulate growth and fat loss not just in your legs but overall. Furthermore, the involvement of some 200 muscles makes the squat one of the most efficient fat burners there is!

Plus, you will be so much better during your next bike ride or soccer match.

16.   More sets are better

If 3 sets of chest exercises are good, then 20 must be great, right? Not quite. The set recommendations for the most effective routine range from Mike Mentzer's high-intensity training (HIT) 1-set routine to Arnold's 25 or more set routine with pretty much every number in between.

So, who is right?

While no one has been able to determine the exact amount of work that it takes to build muscle it seems that between 8 and 12 sets for bigger muscle groups and 6 to 8 sets for smaller groups will do the trick.

The key to building muscle is progression, meaning constant overload with new challenges in weight/intensity. It is simply impossible to perform 20 high-intensity sets for one muscle group and still grow. What matters is how many of your muscle fibers you can hit per session. What does that mean?

As an example, the average trainee can only exhaust about 30% of his muscle fibers in the chest during a set of incline bench press exercises; the second set might add another 10%. So, in order to really get to all the fibers, one would have to perform 5 to 6 sets to the point of muscle failure, which is a recipe for disaster and would lead to overtraining and possibly injury.

Instead, it would be smarter to add exhaustion techniques such as pulses, drop sets or static holds on 2 of your work sets. After that you move on and train the muscle in a stretched position (flyes for chest) to further increase fiber tear. You could then finish up with a pump exercise such as cable crossovers. That's the flexion principle that you find in the works of Holeman and Lawson, which has proven extremely effective.

A note on rep speed: the speed of a repetition matters! Try to be quick and explosive on the positive or concentric phase of the exercise. It doesn't matter if you actually move the weight fast; your body registers the attempt and will recruit more fibers. During the eccentric or negative phase, try to slow down to about 3 seconds. This will increase the workload and muscle damage, which then causes greater adaptations in the muscle.

In terms of time, workouts should be kept short, 45 to 60 minutes including warm up and cool down. After 60 minutes, levels of testosterone tend to drop and cortisol spikes up rather dramatically, which is not a good combination for muscle gain.

You need to set up a plan before you enter the gym, stick to it, hit your muscles intensely and leave. Quality over quantity.

By the same token, training 3 to 4 times a week should be sufficient, provided that you train intensely enough. Any more will most likely not result in greater gains but in overtraining. Remember, you grow outside the gym.

17. A split program is the best way to work out

There is no "one-size-fits-all" program. A spilt program, where you train different body parts over several days in the week, is certainly effective, especially for advanced trainees who can dedicate 4 to 5 hours a week to train. But it is not the be-all and end-all of workout regimens.

There are other ways of training: whole body workouts split by lower body/upper body and push/pull workouts. Bodybuilders often avoid training a muscle several times a week or 2 days in a row, but other athletes do it all the time with great success. Think about speed skaters' or rowers' legs. During the so-called golden age of bodybuilding in the 60's and 70's, guys like Harold Poole would train with whole body workouts all year round. This is probably why they stayed lean even without cardio.

Beginners, especially, should train using whole body workouts at least 3 times per week. Since a beginners' neuro muscular efficiency is not high yet, it makes no sense to focus on one muscle group per day. An all-body workout will elicit a higher response in growth hormone and testosterone. Most beginners would make a lot more progress if they trained with whole body workouts 3 times a week instead of doing 3 days of chest and arms.

Most people have limited time they can dedicate to the gym. When time is of the essence, a whole body routine or a push/pull split workout is a very effective and efficient way to at least maintain strength and size. Whole body workouts are also a great way to stay in shape while traveling since you don't have to worry about missing out on a certain body part for a whole week. Here are some examples of these types of workouts:

Whole body
3 sets x8 reps dead lifts
2x20 leg presses
2 sets of as many pull-ups as you can do
2x12 incline bench presses
2x10 rack pulls
1x10 biceps curls
1 set of as many dips as you can do

Push/Pull

Push day
3x12 squats
1x25 leg presses
3x10 incline barbell bench press
3x15 flat bench dumbbell flyes
3x12 Arnold presses
3x6 close grip bench press
Pull day
Warm up
4x8 dead lifts
3x12 wide grip pull down to the chest
3x10-12 bent over rows
1x10 shrugs
4x10 biceps curl on cable

4x10 straight bar curl
3x8 hammer curls

If you are a beginner, once you complete 1 year to 18 months of training, you should start to split your training into upper body and lower body workouts. Train your weak body parts first, while you still have high energy levels and your concentration is at 100%. I personally believe that one of the most efficient ways to work out is to train your body 3 times in 2 weeks. That split could look some thing like this:

Monday: back and chest
Tuesday: legs and abdominals
Wednesday: off
Thursday: arms, trapezoids, and shoulders
Friday: off
Saturday: restart the cycle with Monday's workout

If you want a simple approach or are time-restricted here is another idea:

Monday: chest/back/shoulders
Wednesday: arms/legs
Friday: whole body workout for power (you could make Friday a high carbohydrate day to really profit from it.)

This type of split workout will enable you to hit your muscles more often with sufficient recovery. You will need to adjust your overall volume in order not to over-train. I recommend 10 to 14 sets for large muscle groups and 6 to 8 for the smaller ones.

To make the workout even more effective, you could create 2 workouts for your chest and alternate between chest workout A and chest workout B. Variety and consistency make for steady gains!

18.   High intensity training (HIT) is the best way to gain mass

In order to better understand HIT, we need a brief history of how it developed.

The science behind HIT

High intensity training is a training technique that was developed in the 70's by Arthur Jones and made popular by the writings of Mike Mentzer. The premise of HIT is to train briefly, intensely, and infrequently. This means you don't train every day in order to allow for maximum recovery. Mike Mentzer even advised his clients to train only once every 6 days.

Because there is an inverse relationship between volume (number of workouts) and intensity (difficulty of workouts), high intensity training sessions are kept short and are usually only comprised of 1 set of 1 exercise per body part. This 1 set is done until total exhaustion of the muscle and is usually followed by static holds or partial repetitions. Other forms of HIT are rest-pause sets and slow negative exercises.

Some HIT protocols call for whole body workouts, others for split training. A common factor is that all HIT trainees use strict form and perform a 4-second negative on each rep. HIT has sparked great controversy within the weightlifting establishment, which advocates a higher volume approach to training, and the 2 camps are deeply divided. Some HIT trainees reported muscle gains of 9 pounds in 14 weeks, but those results should be taken with a big pinch of salt because it is impossible to know how advanced the trainee was and whether or not he took steroids.

What about the real world?

So what are the real life results of HIT training? Jones and Mentzer were certainly correct in their assumption that most people over-train and should work out less frequently or reduce their overall volume. What's more, it is correct that you need to progress in your training to make gains. You need to be able to lift more weight or perform more repetitions during the same time span. Also, I agree with the notion that most people do not need 500 grams of protein a day to grow muscle as was proposed during the 70's.

However, HIT is not the holy grail of muscle building schemes because it does not allow for much flexibility and is simply too dogmatic. Also, there is no scientific proof that one set completed to muscle failure is really all that one needs in order to grow muscle.

Most trainees that went on a HIT program reported good initial gains, which then leveled off. It can be assumed that the initial gains were due to the extra recovery that was possible with a shorter training protocol. In the long run, only very gifted athletes such as Mentzer or Viator continued to make gains. In his book, *The Wisdom of Mike Mentzer*, he says that his best gains came from a 4-day-per-week, multiple-set routine.

I just don't see it...

In my opinion, the problem with HIT is that it can be too rigid and very few trainees have the ability to exhaust their fibers with such low volume. This goes especially for ectomorphs, who tend to have poor recruitment abilities. This means they need to perform a variety of exercises to work their muscles from different positions such as stretched, contracted and mid range to achieve growth. You also need to train more often than once every few days because your ribosome activity (which regulates protein synthesis) declines after 36 hours and your muscles stop adapting. Training to failure at all times will also lead to neural fatigue and might cause injuries (how do you squat to failure anyway?)

However, the idea of spending 4 seconds on the negative part of the repetition is very intriguing. Studies have shown that slowing the negative part of the exercise causes additional muscle damage, which would lead to additional muscle gain and fat loss.

You should definitely look at your overall volume if you haven't made any gains recently. If that were the case, a modified HIT routine would work well for 4 to 6 weeks. Here's an example. The first set should serve as your warm up and the second should be completed to muscle failure:

Workout 1, Monday
2 sets x 10 reps squats
2x12 bench press
2x10 lat pull down
2x10 triceps press downs

Workout 2, Thursday
2x8 dead lifts
2x10 military press
2x10 one arm rows
2x10 barbell curls:

After 6 weeks, I suggest you return to a more volume-oriented approach. The above routine could also be beneficial for someone who is on a strict diet with a severe calorie deficit and who simply doesn't have the energy to go through a traditional split routine.

19.   I want to look like...

This is a double-edged sword. I am a firm believer in visualization, but only up to a certain point.

While it is good to strive for a particular physique, you also have to realize that you are unique. Bodybuilding is a very individual sport; there are no records one can try to break. That also goes for the physiques you see in the magazines. A person that is 6' 2" will never look like David Henry. If your calf insertions are too high, they will never be as big as Mike Matarazzo's.

You need a realistic vision of yourself and what you want to look like, and then you find the strategy to get you there. Do you have body parts you'd like to improve? Do you want to add another 15 pounds of muscle? Drop 2 inches off your waist? Once you know what you want and can achieve, draw up an exercise and nutrition plan for 6 to 12 months. As you go along, you need to have smaller goals that are achievable within a 4-week time frame (upper abs showing, bench up by 5 pounds.) If you fail to achieve those goals, go back to the drawing board and figure out what is wrong. Often it is only a small adjustment that needs to be made, in order to achieve greater results. In my experience, athletes with a poorly laid out plan still do better than those without any plan at all. The steady progress provides motivation to stick with the regiment over the long course.

Another very important tool is visualization; you need to have a vision of what you would like to look like. If that presents a problem, pick someone out of a magazine, or choose Tom Platz's legs, Arnold's biceps, Ronnie's back, and Cutler's haircut as your model. Equipped with these tools, you should reach your potential!

Anyone can build a great physique; it is just a matter of determination and will power. Best of all, it will be yours for the keeping!

20. A wide grip works the outer parts of the muscle

Some muscles, such as the biceps and the quadriceps, have several heads. The theory behind this myth is that by assuming a wide stance/grip, you work the outer head of the muscle.

Actually, the opposite is true. One of the most important rules in training is: out for in, in for out. If you want to build the inner part of your quads, you assume a wide stance for squats and leg presses. If you want to build the outer part of your biceps, you would take a closer grip. Bigger muscles, such as the quads and lats, should be worked from different angles and stances within each workout. Smaller ones, such as the biceps, should be worked with a different grip weekly.

Here are some ideas:

Leg:
Squats: very wide stance for inner thighs, glutes and hamstrings
Leg press: feet wide and high for hamstrings
Leg extensions: feet tilted inward for outer part of the quads

Back:
Rack dead lifts: for the lower back and traps
One-arm rows: for the middle part of the back
Cobras: for the outer lats

Triceps:
Dips: for overall volume
Lying, overhead dumbbell extensions: for the inner head
Rope extensions at the cable: outer head

Biceps:
Narrow grip pull-ups: outer head
Wide grip barbell curls: inner head
Thick grip hammer curls: forearm and brachioradialis

21.   Squats give you a big butt

There is some truth to this. Because the squat is a functional leg exercise it involves the glutes, hamstrings, quadriceps, and even calves.

Now, some people won't mind building up their rear end or making it a little firmer. However, trainees with short legs can develop a blocky physique if they focus too much on the back squat. For trainees with shorter legs, it would make sense to switch temporarily to front squats to stress the quadriceps more.

In order to achieve a symmetrical leg development, leg presses with the feet wide and low would de-emphasize the workload of the glutes.

Also hack squats and sissies are a good addition for proper quad development.

If glutes are one of your weaker points, I would definitely add walking lunges and stiff legged dead lifts in order to train the muscle from all angles.

Sometimes a change in diet and reduction in body fat can also cause a significant reduction in the size of your bum since not all size is muscle.

22.   You can alter the shape of your muscles by performing certain exercises

Some exercises are often called "shaping exercises." Cable concentration curl for the biceps peak is one. Unfortunately, the shape of a muscle is genetically determined and no exercise will alter it. But that doesn't mean that your physique is predetermined. You need to look at yourself the way an artist would and decide where do you need more or less "clay", as Arnold put it in *Pumping Iron*.

So if your biceps don't have much of a peak, you should first try to increase the overall mass in your arm. After that, work on the brachioradialis, which will push your biceps up more. I would recommend reverse or Zottman curls. If your quads lack sweep, it is necessary to build more mass on the outer part of the muscle. The weapon of choice would be the close stance squat or leg extensions with outward pointed toes. If your lats are too high, you need to work the insertions to make them seem wider. You should start doing high rep V handle pull downs to the chest where you sit almost upright.

Lacking shoulder width can be corrected with leaning side raises. My favorite workout would be the following:

Warm up thoroughly with a few light sets then grab a dumbbell, which is about 120% of your regular training weight and perform 5 to 6 repetitions, using your body if needed, then drop the weight by 50% for another 10 slow, very strict repetitions. Two sets of this combination should ignite new growth.

Bodybuilding is about creating a physique that works for you. You need to get an understanding of anatomy and how muscles function. That combined with a proper nutritional program will be the ticket to your dream body.

23. Women should not lift weights because it will make them bulky

Wrong, wrong, wrong! Women do not posses enough testosterone to build large amounts of muscle. Just to give you an idea, a healthy young male produces about 6 to 11 milligrams a day or 45 to 80 milligrams per week. Women manufacture about a quarter of a milligram per day. Too often, women are held back from lifting because they get freaked out by pictures of female bodybuilders in magazines. Women do not bulk up like that naturally. Those athletes have used steroids (male hormones) to achieve an extraordinary amount of muscle. Dosages here can range from 50 to 150 milligrams per week, so it is obvious where the extra muscle mass comes from.

For the natural trainee, this simply won't happen. Every pound of muscle a natural athlete puts on (which can be a struggle) will significantly speed up the metabolism, thereby making fat loss easier. And since muscle has much less volume than fat, there will be a reduction in overall size.

If you started training with weights and noticed an increase in size, check your diet. Chances are it isn't muscle…

Weight training in combination with a proper nutritional protocol is the fastest and most effective way to achieve the physique you want.

24.   Low repetitions are for bulking

This is a gray area as there is some truth to it. In the 60's, bodybuilders used to compete also as weightlifters and often trained liked them during the winter. They would focus on the squat, dead lift, and bench, drop their repetitions to 3 to 5 and perform more sets to work on their strength. This went hand in hand with an increased food intake and yielded a considerable increase in muscle mass. The question remains whether it was the low repetitions or the food intake that caused the surge in mass.

As I've mentioned before, nobody has established the perfect rep number that would make everyone grow. While 8 to 12 repetitions seems like a good range to agree on, there is also Bill Starr's 5x5, Rory Leidelmeyers 100 repetitions, and Vince Gironda's 8x8—systems that have been proven to build muscle mass.

I personally would not train with really low repetitions (below 3), as it results in a higher creatinine and cortisol output, thereby causing muscle loss and mental fatigue. Such low rep numbers serve mainly to improve the neural drive to the muscle without causing much hypertrophy (muscle gain) which makes them an interesting choice for athletes, such as wrestlers and swimmers, who want to improve their strength without gaining mass. For a physique athlete, I don't see the need to train with such low repetitions since the risk of injury increases exponentially.

Then there is food intake. Without a calorie surplus, no training system will build muscle. It wasn't uncommon back then to consume a gallon of milk and several dozen eggs on a daily basis. I think this is overkill, but if your goal is to bulk up, you need to eat. So take your BMR and add 500 calories per day to it. This should yield a relatively clean weekly gain of half a pound of muscle.

But that still doesn't answer the question of whether low repetitions (3 to 6) build more mass than higher repetitions.

I believe the answer lies in your body type. Mesomorphs will definitely grow on low repetitions as well as heavy weights since they have the bone structure and fiber type for it. But even if you fall into that category you should perform some higher rep sets to fully exhaust the type 2 fibers.

Ectomorphs, on the other hand, will most likely get nothing out of it since they have lower neural output (ability to activate muscle fibers) and are simply not capable of exhausting their fibers during a low-volume workout. They have fewer fast twitch fibers, meaning they need to train at a higher volume in order to get to the endurance oriented fibers. They should try to get a pump in every workout, keep their repletion numbers higher and use stretching exercises for each muscle to expand muscle volume: sissies, incline curls, flyes.

Furthermore, not all muscles are created equal. Because the quadriceps are much more of an endurance muscle than the hamstrings, the training should be adjusted accordingly. Sets on the leg press can be up to 30 repetitions whereas the leg curl and the dead lift should be kept around 8. Calf and forearm training is also very endurance based. Repetitions can easily go into the 25 and above range.

Some people also might require a hybrid method, where you would perform 2 to 3 low rep power sets in the range of 5 to 8 repetitions and then add some high rep pump work for each muscle group. The 21-system would be a good follow up.

So there you have it, no easy answer on this one. You will need to experiment and see what works for you. But remember; give every training system 6 weeks to prove itself. It is crucial to keep a diary and take pictures at the beginning and the end of each 6- to 8-week training cycle.

If you have a lot of pain tolerance, try to train with 100s for a week or 10 days, it will be a welcome shock for your body. Pick one or at most two exercises per body part and use about 50% of your regular weight, 60% if you are more ambitious. This will allow you to perform up to 50 repetitions, rest 1 second for every rep you are missing to 100. Perform as many sets as needed to get to 100 repetitions. The pain will be brutal, but chances you initiate new growth!

25. You need a pump for muscles to grow

This is mostly true. While there are some people that can grow on very low repetitions due to their high neuromuscular efficiency, the rest of us should try to get a pump.

A pump should be achieved by moving heavy weights for 8-12 reps, not by doing cable flyes with 20 pounds for 25 or more sets. The effect is that you shuttle additional blood to your target muscle. This achieves two things: you reached your target muscle (which may always not be the case with your back or hamstrings since they are out of sight) and the target muscle gets more nutrients via the increased blood flow. These elements in combination ensure muscle growth.

There is also empirical evidence that a pump might be able to stretch the fascia (a sock-like tissue surrounding the muscle). This is significant because the fascia, when tight, constricts the muscle from expanding. If you can stretch it, there is more room for the muscle to grow. I remain skeptical of the relation between the stretching of the fascia and the growth of a muscle. If I were not, however, I would prefer to use stretch exercises, such as sissy squats or dumbbell flyes rather than a pump to create the intended effect.

Studies on birds have shown a 300% increase in muscle mass when they worked against a stretch resistance. While this is certainly not one to one applicable to humans, it still shows the potential.

Lastly, getting a pump feels great and makes for a more productive workout! What a shame it only lasts 20 minutes.

26. You need to go to failure on every set during every workout

Doing this is the quickest way to burn out and put a screeching halt to your gains. You maybe even be setting yourself up for an injury. If you push your muscles constantly to failure, you will experience fatigue.

There are two types of fatigue: muscular and mental. Your muscles actually recover rather quickly and can be worked within 48 hours of your last session. If you look at speed skaters or rowers, you will find that they squat up to 12 times a week without overtraining their legs. Now this seems to go against any conventional wisdom since it screams overtraining. And yet these athletes have a large amount of muscle mass. What's the story here?

First, speed skaters and rowers are superior conditioned full-time professional athletes. Second, they have a better ability to recover than most people. But hardly any of these sessions are done to failure in order to avoid mental exhaustion. An interesting approach regarding the idea of more frequent but less intense training would be Bryan Hancock's HST (Hypertrophy Specific Training) program.

So does this mean you can and should train 12 times a week?

Not at all, but you should be aware that there is an inverse relationship between volume and intensity. If you train with a high intensity your volume needs to decrease. It is impossible to train intensely all year round, which is why it would be a good idea to schedule weeks off and/or weeks where you only train with 70% of your usual weights without forced repetitions.

This will accomplish two things: first, it will allow your joints and ligaments to heal, and second, it will enable you to recharge and make greater gains upon your return to training.

Also, you should not perform more than 1 or 2 sets to failure per exercise and keep the number of exercises per muscle group between 3 and 5. Twenty or more all-out sets of curls will not give you bigger arms but most likely an inflamed elbow. So cycle your intensity, give your body a chance to recover and grow. You will be surprised how much quicker you make progress.

27. Ab blaster, ab roller, ab wheel, the super ab machine

No other muscle suggests as many gadgets and gizmos than the abdominal muscles. Remember the movie *Something About Mary*, when the hitchhiker convinces Ben Stiller's character that 6-minute abs is the way to go, as opposed to 7-minute abs? You save 1 minute, after all.

Then there are ab blasters, trimmers, shapers, benches... Do these contraptions work? Well some of them will cause your abs to contract and relax, i.e., train them, but they are no more efficient than the knee up or the leg raise. If you want to really involve your entire core, then exercises such as the squat, dead lift, or overhead press deliver the most for your money.

No device or training system will give you visible abs if your body fat percentage is not at least 10%. So in addition to training your abs once or twice a week, you would need to shed those pounds.

28. Electro stimulation helps to grow muscle

Electro stimulation was big in the 90's; many gyms offered it on the side to make your pectorals bigger and your abs more cut at the same time. Electro stimulation is a great tool to rehab injured trainees, but it will do very little if anything to build muscle and burn fat.

If you are looking to optimize your training, visualize before you work out. Go through the motion in your head so that you feel a slight contraction and relaxation of your target muscles. This will improve your neural output and activate a higher number of fibers during your training, which will lead to greater gains.

29. Bodybuilders aren't really strong

It is often said that "bodybuilders are not as strong as they look." That statement is partly envy (or so I tell myself), but it also contains a morsel of truth.

Bodybuilding is a sport where only appearance matters. How you got your physique is of no interest unless you want to wear a "400-Pound Squat" T-shirt at the beach.

So, are bodybuilders a bunch of weaklings? Not at all. First, anyone with above average muscle mass has above average strength. But in general, physique athletes are not as strong as power lifters because strength is simply not on the focus of their training programs.

We need to look at the difference between training for strength and training for hypertrophy in order to understand the two approaches. Strength training—the type that power lifters prefer—is done with a higher set and lower rep volume, the famous "5x5" or "4-4-3-3-2-2" rep patterns. This type of training increases neuromuscular efficiency, which allows the lifting of heavier weights, but it does not build a lot of mass because the growth hormone output and muscle fiber recruitment are limited.

Hypertrophy training tends to follow a higher reps/fewer sets pattern. Here the focus is on gaining quality mass; any strength gain is an added bonus.

So the main difference is that bodybuilders perform most of their repetitions in the 80 to 85% range, whereas power lifters train mostly in the 90 to 95% range.

Should bodybuilders include some strength training in their regime? I believe so; in fact, a hybrid training approach would yield great benefits for both groups. The stronger you are as a bodybuilder, the more weight you can move in your hypertrophy workouts, which will lead to greater gains.

Beginners especially should focus on getting stronger, since strength precedes muscle mass. I would, however, stay away from heavy singles or doubles since the risk of injury rises dramatically without much added benefit.

A good 4-week strength cycle would look like this:

Monday:
Heavy squat: 5 sets x 5 reps squat
Medium bench: 5x5 incline bench press
Row: 5x5 bent over rows

Wednesday:
Heavy bench: 5x5 incline bench press
Medium row: 5x5 bent over row (60% of Friday's heavy set)
Light squat: 5x5 front squat (40 to 50% of Monday's weight)

Friday:
Heavy row: 5x5 bent over row
Medium squat: 5x5 squat (60% of Monday's heavy set)
Light bench: 5x5 military press

Whereby heavy means 85 to 90% of the maximum training weight, medium is about 70%, and light 40 to 50%.

You can add arm and other auxiliary exercises as you see fit as long as you progress every week. Try to increase the weights 3 to 5% per week on your heavy days.

Arnold got his tremendous base from a high amount of strength training in his early years. He was known for benching

500 pounds, and his training partner, Franco Columbo, dead lifted 700 or more pounds. Not bad for someone who only "looks" strong.

30. You need to stretch before lifting weights

Stretching is something many people just do because they feel they should or someone told them to. Stretching is supposed to prevent injuries by elongating the muscle. Does it really?

The opposite is true. Stretching before lifting weights weakens the muscle by up to 30%. What's more, it also increases the risk of injury because there is less tension in the muscle. You don't want to go under a heavy squat with loose quadriceps!

The pro-stretching advocates will say that stretching makes a muscle more malleable. How would that work? You can't make a rubber band more flexible! In order to gain flexibility, you need to change the structure of a muscle, by stretching it through the full range of motion with weights. In other words, you need to develop strength around the joint, not just flexibility.

This does not mean you should not warm up. During warm up, more is actually better. Perform 3 to 5 light warm-up sets to get blood into muscles and ligaments and sharpen your form; then work your way up to training weight.

So does stretching have no place in weight training? It certainly does, but *after* you train. As mentioned before, stretching can help by breaking up the fascia. Weighted stretches or static stretches could be done with certain exercises, such as incline curls for your biceps, flyes for the chest or dumbbell pullovers for your lats.

Static stretches should be held for 30 to 45 seconds to have an effect. You can statically stretch every muscle group after you are done training that particular body part.

31. Weightlifting stunts growth so kids shouldn't lift weights

For a long time it was believed that training with weights would prematurely close the epiphyseal growth plates in the long bones of the body, thereby stunting growth. It was for that reason that kids were not encouraged to train with weights, but rather to play sports instead.

But consider this: while playing sports is undoubtedly good for kids, during a basketball game there are forces working on the knees and ankles that are several times the kid's bodyweight.

Therefore, it might actually be a good idea for teenagers to train with weights in order to prevent sports injuries. There is absolutely nothing to the growth-stunting myth. As long as you lift with good form and adequate rest, nothing bad will happen. Some studies such as the Russian school of height even suggest that training with weights spurs growth. In any event, it allows teens to grow up with stronger ligaments and muscles.

Steroids, on the other hand, are known to stunt growth, so nobody should touch them before at least 21 years of age (after that, they are still illegal but at least you will be your maximum height when facing the jury).

32. Isometrics build muscle

Remember Charles Atlas and his program? He incorporated some self-resistance exercises, such as pitting one limb against the other, to maximize muscular output. While he was certainly a pioneer in physical exercise, things have changed a bit since then.

There are three ways a muscle can perform work: concentrically, which is pushing or pulling and decreasing the joint angle); eccentrically, which is the negative part of the repetition, lowering weight against a resistance thereby increasing the joint angle; and finally, isometrically, which is a static hold where the joint angle doesn't change. If you want to change your body, you will need to engage as many muscle fibers as possible. The concentric and eccentric phases are your bread and butter in that regard.

The concentric, or negative, part of an exercise is often wasted due to sloppy form. Yet your muscles can actually perform the most work during that movement. Try to devote 1 to 2 sets per exercise where you give the negative part 2 to 3 seconds; you will be sore the next day!

What about isometrics? A study from NASA has shown that they fail to prevent the breakdown of contractile proteins, which cause the muscle to degrade and lose strength. So as a form of training in itself, isometrics are not very helpful. An exception would be physical rehabilitation—helping someone recovering from an injury to relearn functional muscle movements. They could also be a good add-on to a weight-lifting routine. Once you have completed a set to the point where you simply cannot move the weight another inch, try and perform a static hold for 15 seconds. Good exercises for this technique would be leg extensions, pectoral dec, pullovers, and concentration curls.

Another way to use isometrics, according to Bill Star, would be to implement them as a light workout during the week, almost as an active recovery. Find a rack and lock the bar in a position of overhead presses, 3 sets of 12 seconds, then do the same with rows and squats. Press the bar as hard as you can for each repetition. The whole workout should not take more than 15 minutes. This would be a good way to keep your strength levels up if you perform in a sport on the weekends and don't want to fatigue your CNS. Just don't expect too much muscle growth from it.

33.   You can reduce body fat in a spot

I am sorry, but spot reduction does not work. Have you ever seen someone doing 500 or more twists in order to get pronounced obliques? It never happens.

In short, if your body fat percentage is too high, your abs will not be visible. If your overall body fat is 20% and you are doing hundreds of crunches a day, your body will still not give you a midsection that is at 8% body fat and leave the rest at 20%.

So if you want visible muscles, you first need to determine how many pounds you will need to lose. As an example: for a 200 pound athlete with 20% body fat, in order to see abs, 10% body fat would be a good goal. Since that person currently holds 40 pounds of fat, he would need to drop about 25 pounds of fat to get to 175 pounds, at which point he would be around 8% with great abs. Keep in mind that this is a hypothetical example since some muscle mass would be lost as well during the diet.

In order to lose 25 pounds, a 20-week diet would be appropriate to drop about 1 to 1.5 pounds a week, which would enable the trainee to hold on to most of his muscle. Since a pound of fat holds 3,500 calories, in order to lose 1 pound per week, you need to create a 500-calorie deficit per day.

Part of this deficit (80%) should be created through limted calorie intake and the rest through exercise. Which kind of exercise?

The best way to understand this is to imagine your fat deposits as a gigantic fuel storage facility. Your job is to burn all this fuel ASAP. For that task, you are given two tools: a lawn mower and a jet fighter. Sure, both have combustible engines, but which one will go through the fuel faster?

It's all about energy expenditure

Doing crunches is the equivalent of the lawn mower since it burns very few calories, (20 minutes of crunches burns about 50 calories, which means one would have to do 3.5 hours of crunches a day to expend the 500 calories). So you need to deploy the big multi-joint exercises (your F-14 fighter plane), such as the squat, dips, pull downs, dead lifts, and shoulder press as well as a strict diet to burn a sufficient amount of energy. The weight lifting will enable you to hold on to your muscles and prevent the metabolic rate from dropping while some added cardio could help with creating an additional energy deficit.

You can still throw in some crunches twice a week to show off your abs, but you will need to make them visible first.

34. Go heavy or go home

Lifting heavy builds bigger muscles, right? It's true that if you put more stress on your muscles, consume enough calories, and rest accordingly, your muscles will show signs of hypertrophy.

But it is not so much about the numbers on the bar as the actual amount of work you put on the muscle. A runner's squat (2-inch movement of the knees) will put most of the strain on the knee, and you will not experience much leg improvement. Take 40 to 50% of the weight off and squat deep for 10 to 15 repetitions, and very soon you will see your legs getting leaner and more muscular (plus you save yourself from an ACL surgery).

Somebody who performs a curl with 100 pounds but swings wildly up and down on each rep (every gym has one of these guys) is stressing his biceps with only 30 pounds; the rest is being moved by his lower back, momentum, etc. The elbows, however, are taking the full 100 pounds as an impact. So this trainee is setting himself up for an injury without having trained his target muscle properly.

A better approach would be to periodize your training. As an example you could perform 2 weeks with sets of 15, 2 weeks with sets of 10, and 2 weeks with sets of 5 with increasing weights. This would be Bryan Haycock's HST system. Another approach would be to train 2 weeks for power with 6 to 8 repetitions, 2 weeks for hypertrophy with 8 to 12 repetitions, and then shock the body with 2 weeks of drop sets—pulses to stimulate new growth.

Bodybuilding is not weight lifting. So, while it is nice to set new records, you always have to try to engage the most fibers in order to force a change in your body. You should always strive for progress, be it more weight or more repetitions. But never forego good form so you stay injury free and achieve maximum results.

35. Once you stop training all the muscle will turn into fat

Since muscle and fat are two entirely different entities, one cannot simply become the other. If someone with an above average muscle mass stops training altogether—perhaps because of an injury—yet continues eating the same amount of calories, he will quickly build an unsightly layer of fat. The muscle, on the other hand, will slowly be broken down since it is not needed anymore.

So does that mean you can't take even a 2-week vacation? Not at all! Muscle loss doesn't start for about 10 days in the case of total inactivity. Most trainees should take a week off every 10 to 12 weeks. Because they are most likely over-trained, there is a good chance they might actually grow during the r rest period.

During that period, I recommend maintaining high protein intake but lowering your carbohydrate consumption since your act vity level is less.

If you want to engage in other activities, that's fine as long as the total volume is kept below 5 hours a week.

The good news for bodybuilder X is that once he starts training and eating right again, muscle memory kicks in, which will enable him to regain the mass rather quickly.

36. You have to eat big to get big

The traditional bodybuilding cycle goes something like this: eat like a horse during the cold months, then diet during spring and summer to show off some abs.

Now, to be clear, in order to build muscle you have to consume more energy than you need. The question is how much mcre and what kind?

Basically, there are two types of bulking: the dirty bulk where anything goes, including junk food, and the clean bulk, where the vast majority of your calories comes from clean foods only. The dirty bulk leads to greater mass gains, but most of it is fat and water, which then need to be dieted off. Since the diet has to be a lot longer, most of the newly gained muscle mass will also be lost. What happens often is that the athlete eats like a horse for 16 weeks, diets very strictly for 20 weeks and looks the same as he did 36 weeks before.

As you can tell, I am a fan of the clean bulk, since that tends to keep athletes lean year round while providing steady gans. Keep in mind that there will always be a certain amount of fat gained when trying to pack on muscle.

However, in a clean bulk you should be able to gain two-thirds muscle and one-third fat. If you do this correctly, you should still be fairly lean since your body fat percentage is not going up exponentially.

A good starting point for any mass-gaining diet would be to eat 2-3 grams of carbohydrates from good carbohydrate sources, such as oats, brown rice, and potatoes for every pound of bodyweight and one gram of protein per pound of bodyweight. It would be preferable to choose rather lean protein sources such as chicken, whey protein, lean beef, and fish. As for the fats, these will be provided with your eggs and beef; in addition, you should consume nuts, avocados, and olive oil as well as fish oil capsules.

After 5 days of eating a high-carbohydrate/low-fat approach, double your protein and cut your carbohydrates in half while adding substantially more healthy fats to the diet. This will result in temporary overfeeding, which causes a burst of anabolic hormones. These will help with recovery as well as muscle growth without gaining a lot of body fat, since the time span is simply too short for your body to store it.

Someone who is carbohydrate sensitive—meaning does not react well to carbohydrates and gets bloated very fast—should turn the above pattern around: Monday to Friday you would eat high protein, medium fat, and low carbohydrates, and during the weekend switch to a high carbohydrate, medium protein, low fat eating pattern. The two carbohydrate days serve to restore the glycogen in the muscle and keep the thyroid running.

By changing your intake, your body will not get stuck in a rut, and the gains will keep coming. Even when bulking, I would still perform 2 to 3 cardio sessions a week to ensure optimal digestion and oxidization of the muscles. There you have it, a way to get bigger without expanding your waistline too much!

37.   Free weights are better than machines

There are some eternal debates: Yankees versus Red Sox, BMW versus Mercedes, and free weights versus machines. It has been said that training with free weights builds more muscle than machines. The truth lies somewhere in between and depends on a variety of factors, such as training goals, experience, and coordination.

Free weights are excellent because they adapt to the natural movements of the body. What's more, training with free weights engages the stabilizing muscles and teaches balance. Someone training for a specific sport would do well to include lots of free weight exercise into their training program, since dumbbells and barbells offer excellent ways to simulate certain movements.

Machines, on the other hand, force the athlete into a certain movement without allowing for much flexibility. On the plus side, one can usually use more weight on machines since there is no balance to worry about. More weight leads to a greater activation of fibers within the target muscle, which makes for better gains.

Beginners usually do better with machines since their overall coordination is not very well developed. Machine training in this context is a good way to gain muscle awareness before moving on to free weights. Someone coming back from an injury would also benefit from a machine-based approach as it allows him to regain stability before returning to free weights.

What about the advanced trainee? I am afraid there is no easy answer. In order to achieve maximum results you must target the muscle fully. A lot of people are stuck in their belief that you need to load a lot of weight on a barbell and then perform quarter repetitions for the bench or squat. This form of training will get you nowhere but to the ER. You need to go through the full range of motion while trying to properly activate your target muscle. If a machine helps you to achieve that, then by all means use it. If you need dumbbells or a barbell to feel the muscle working, go for it.

When structuring a workout, I would perform free weight exercises first since they require more coordination. In general, you get more for your money with free weights since they include more muscles and cause a higher activation of fibers.

Machines would be used later in the workout to fully exhaust the muscle. They can be a great tool for intensity techniques, such as drop sets or pulses, since it is easy to change weights and the risk of an injury is lower than when there is a 300-pound barbell dangling over your head.

Then there is the matter of different muscles reacting to different styles of training. In my case, dumbbells work great for my biceps, but I have a hard time using them for my hamstrings, which is why I resort to the leg curl. So, it is good to mix free weights and machines for maximal results. But make sure you feel the muscle working— Don't just move weight around!

38. Ab- and adductor machines are great for slimming thighs

Abductor and adductor machines are in high-demand in any gym, primarily by women, but the question remains whether it makes sense to use them.

Let's look at the anatomy. Both are small muscles. The adductor's function is to pull your knee inwards over the midline, whereas the abductors move it outward. Since a lot of fat is stored on the inner thigh, using the abductor machines seems like a great idea. It isn't.

The adductor muscles are too small to use up much energy (i.e., stored fat) when worked by themselves. You are much better off training your legs with big compound movements such as squats and walking lunges. These will engage all muscles and not just the relatively small ad/abductors.

There may be some cases where you need to work on your adductors directly in order to prevent an injury or discomfort. For example, if your knees buckle inward while squatting, you have weak abductors. If untreated, it can lead to problems with the knees and hips.

A good way to correct this is to perform bodyweight squats with a resistance band wrapped around the knees as a warm-up before training legs. This will strengthen your abductors and enable you to perform proper squats.

If your goal is fat loss in the thigh area, your best exercises are the squat using different stances, lunges, step-ups (vertical and horizontal) as well as the leg press. Once you have achieved sufficient leanness but are stuck with some stubborn fat deposits, a topical cream with caffeine, yohimbe, and aminophylline can make the difference.

Oh, and did I mention that fat loss is 80% diet?

39. Weight training makes you stiff and inflexible

This myth has been around forever. In the past, coaches told their athletes not to lift weights because it would make them stiff.

That is simply not true. Being overly bulky makes you stiff, but training with weights does not. If you have ever seen the muscular frames of gymnasts, you will see that they move quite a bit of weight, and yet they are extremely flexible.

Weight training with proper form and the full range of motion actually increases flexibility since it moves muscles, joints, and ligaments through the whole range of motion. If you have performed a deep fly motion for the pectorals, you will understand that it would be very hard to achieve such a deep stretch any other way than with dumbbells. The same goes for incline curls for biceps and sissy squats for the quadriceps. I would perform a stretch exercise for every muscle after training it with a big compound movement, to ensure blood flow, recovery, and flexibility.

Here are my favorites for each muscle:

Quads: sissy squats
Hamstrings: stiff legged dead lifts
Calves: donkey raises
Lats: dumbbell pullovers
Mid back: rope rows or one-arm rows with dumbbells
Pecs: Dumbbell flyes
Shoulders: leaning side rises
Traps: dumbbell shrugs
Biceps: incline curls
Triceps: one arm overhead extensions seated or standing

Add 2 to 3 sets of a stretch exercise after you finish your heavy work and you will soon realize new growth, strength, and better blood flow in your muscles. And as for static stretches, always perform these AFTER the workout!

40. Cheat repetitions are good for muscle growth

Everyone who has ever been to a gym has seen cheat repetitions performed, mostly by a group of overly motivated teenagers trying to curl 100 or more pounds. At times, the barbell curl reminds you more of a limbo dance "how low can I go?" That is one side of the spectrum. On the other hand, you see bodybuilding greats like Arnold or Ronnie Coleman losing their form during the last repetitions of a set and it seems to work just fine for them.

So are cheat repetitions dangerous or muscle building? Probably both. The truth is most people use them incorrectly. If you need to swing your lower back from the first rep of you set of curls, then the weight is too heavy. However, cheat repetitions if used properly can be very helpful for your progress since they allow you to fully fatigue a muscle. Let's assume you are curling 60 pounds. During the first 7 repetitions, you are perfectly capable of moving 60 pounds, but then your strength drops to 50 pounds. So the set is over?

Not quite, if you involve your delts and lower back just enough for the last rep, you will be able to exhaust the fibers in your target muscle even further. Make sure you do it in a controlled fashion to avoid injuries. You can also recruit other muscle groups. For instance, you can use your legs, when doing standing shoulder presses, just push off lightly or press your hands on your thighs when performing leg presses.

Here are my favorite cheat moves:

Legs: leg press, hands help on thighs
Back: cable pull downs/rows with a slight tilt from the upper body going backwards or single arm cable rows where the free hand supports the pulling
Chest: dumbbell flyes, which turn into presses as you fatigue
Shoulder: standing press, dumbbells or barbell, where you use your legs to achieve lift off
Arms: single arm curls or triceps extensions where you use your free hand to support you

Reserve cheat repetitions for your last set and don't perform them on every exercise. Otherwise you might over-train.

Part II
Cardio

41.   Cardio at a target heart rate burns only fat—there is a fat burning zone

When it comes to cardio advice in the fitness industry, it is really a case of the blind leading the blind. Statements that have no scientific background are being recapitulated without regard to their validity. Case in point, the fat burning zone.

On a lot of cardio equipment, you find graphs telling you which heart rate you should be in for cardiovascular or fat burning training. They usually determine these by subtracting your age from 200 beats per minute for cardio and 60% of that number for maximum fat loss. The logic behind it is that training at a lesser intensity will use primarily fat for energy, while training at a higher intensity uses glycogen (carbohydrates.) Sounds great and seems very scientific, but it is not accurate!

The body's energy system is too complex to be fooled by a simple number of heartbeats. The only time when you burn fats exclusively is when you are asleep. The drawback is that when you sleep you are not terribly active, so your overall energy consumption is low. During all other times your body uses fat *and* carbohydrates for energy. It is true that during low-intensity cardio more calories are derived from fat than during high intensity interval training (HIIT), but the overall number of calories burned is also much lower.

So in the end you would still be better off performing interval training, especially since excess post-exercise consumption (EPOC) or oxygen debt is much higher with high-intensity than with low-intensity cardio. This is called the "after burn effect" and it accounts for another 50 calories burned in the 24 hours after the cardio session, which doesn't seem like a lot, but it can be for athletes who are already very lean and for whom every little bit counts. There is some research that this type of cardio workout is a more effective way to burn fat. So is low intensity cardio useless? No, there are two instances when it is perfect: after a workout with weights and during a low-carbohydrate diet. After training with weights, your glycogen stores are depleted and there are more free form fatty acids in your bloodstream. Low- to medium-intensity cardio is a good way to burn them off.

Anyone on a low carbohydrate diet is by definition glycogen depleted and any HIIT cardio would lead to muscle loss. Training at about one 100 to 120 beats per minute (BPM) would be a good way to lose fat without sacrificing muscle. Since most people can perform medium intensity cardio for a longer period of time than HIIT, they end up buring the same number of calories.

I would advise you to chose according to your personal preference. If you are pressed for time, perform HIIT cardio. If you have the time and your resistance workouts are already very demanding, stick with medium intensity cardio. Also, don't fall for the myth that it takes 20 minutes for the body to start tapping into the fat storage. Energy production is a 24 hour cycle; there is no magic switch your body turns on after 20 minutes to burn fat for energy. What matters is the overall intake versus the overall energy expenditure.

I also find it crucial to vary your cardio between the bike, treadmill, and Stairmaster. During summer, try to incorporate as much outdoor cardio as possible. It is more fun and the added sun exposure will help you achieve better definition.

42. Cardio is to get lean; weightlifting is to bulk up

Anyone who has ever worked out in a gym has noticed that there is without fail a certain group of treadmill addicts that spend hours every day running—yet they never get lean. On the other hand, you have people with great abs and overall lean physiques that never set foot on any cardio equipment but move a considerable amount of iron on the gym floor.

This seems to go against anything you have ever read or heard, but why? Most importantly, your body composition depends on your diet. Any form of training can only help to create a calorie deficit. Most people take it as gospel that weight lifting is exclusively to get bigger. But the truth is that while weight lifting can create bigger muscles, it can also create a leaner physique, depending on dietary factors.

Cardio and weightlifting burn about the same amount of calories, but resistance training will help you to hold on to your muscle. When you diet, the body wants to cannibalize unused muscle for energy; training with weights prevents that from happening. In addition, it keeps your basic metabolic rate (BMR) elevated since it uses energy to repair the damage from your last weight workout. As for the bulking part, only resistance training combined with a calorie surplus will build additional muscle mass.

Cardio is very useful as a supplemental energy expenditure in order to create an even bigger calorie deficit. Cardio can also be used to burn off free fatty acids, which occur in greater concentration in your blood stream after lifting weights.

In short then, lifting weights can get you very lean if you eat properly. I am even going out on a limb when I say that most males can get lean without doing any cardio. The reason is that someone who weighs 200 pounds and has a maintenance caloric need of 3,000 calories a day can easily create a 1,500 calorie deficit, which will be enough to lose up to 4 pounds a week. Add to the mix 3 weight-training sessions to preserve muscle and you won't need any cardio. Cardio can help to speed up the process (especially in smaller individuals and women), but cardio alone will not get you the physique you desire.

If your goal is to get leaner, the most important thing is to outline the appropriate diet to fit your needs. In order to lose a pound of body fat you will need to create a 3,500-calorie deficit. Stretched over a week that means you will need to create a deficit of 500 calories per day of which 80% has to come from your diet, the rest from exercise.

You will need to log your calories, at least for the first 3 weeks, to get a clear picture of how many calories you are taking in. I actually prefer to get a weekly balance since there are always day-to-day swings and you don't burn the same amount of calories every day. A weekly approach will also allow you a little more sophisticated dieting with high and low days.

One way to approach it is to follow a zigzag calorie count over the course of the week. Let's assume your daily calorie goal is 1500 calories. From there you could break down your week as follows: Monday 1500, Tuesday 1300, Wednesday 1500, Thursday 1300, Friday 1700, Saturday 1700 and Sunday 1500. This would allow you to go out with friends on the weekends while keeping your metabolism guessing so it doesn't stall out on you.

43. Don't do cardio when you're trying to bulk up

When someone is trying to put on weight, cardio seems like a bad idea since it is extra energy expenditure. In fact, it should still be done for several reasons. First, it keeps you heart healthy and provides an overall sense of well-being. Second, it shuttles oxygen to you muscles. The better oxygenated they are, the better they can grow. This will also help with recovery after workouts. Performing some low-intensity cardio right after training legs will reduce soreness the day after.

Lastly, cardio helps with digestion, which is not to be taken lightly when you're taking in 5,000 or more calories per day to bulk up. A good guideline is this: 3 30-minute sessions per week at a low to medium intensity. It's also going to keep you lean enough to have your abs visible even when bulking. Remember, it's called body building not belly building!

If you are an extreme hard gainer or work in a profession that involves a lot of physical activity, such as a bike courier, dock worker, or farm hand, you can skip the cardio altogether.

44. Should cardio be done before or after weightlifting?

It's not uncommon to see people running on the treadmill for 30 minutes or more in order to achieve some fat loss before lifting. This is not a good idea for several reasons. First, cardio lowers your testosterone levels and spikes cortisol, which is not a good way to start a weights workout.

Consider this: If you start the workout with lower levels of your muscle-building hormones, you will be at a significant disadvantage from the start. Training with weights also requires more concentration than cardio, so it should be done first. Very little can happen on a stationary bike, but a 300 pound bench press or squat is a different matter.

Lastly, cardio after weights is a much more effective fat burner than before. Weight training exhausts the glycogen stores in the muscle, therefore requiring the body to free up fatty acids for energy production. These fatty acids are much more prevalent in your blood stream after lifting, so if you perform 15 to 20 minutes of cardio after your weight training (without going over 60 to 70 minutes of total training time) you have added an excellent fat burning tool to your arsenal.

45. Wearing warm-ups while doing cardio burns more fat

One can still see people running on the treadmill in sweats or even plastic wrap. This is a bad idea, which at best is ineffective and at worst lethal since it can lead to severe dehydration and heat stroke. More sweating does not equal more fat loss. The extra weight you drop is water and will come back right after you consume liquids. If there were any truth to it, you wouldn't have to diet just sit in the sauna and walk out lean. There is no fat in sweat.

It is actually counterproductive to be dressed in several layers since your output is diminished. Research has shown that a cooler environment forces the body to work harder to create energy. In a study in the journal of *Medicine and Science in Sports and Exercise*, it was found that the caloric expenditure was 13% higher in a colder environment. This might be why cardio in the morning seems to be more effective since your core temperature is lower.

Once you are dehydrated, the body stops fat loss in order to conserve water, which is another reason not to wrap yourself up like a sausage.

As for building muscle, there is some evidence to support a connection between warmth and growth (maybe that's why California is the Mecca of bodybuilding). If your core temperature is higher, you will have better blood flow and fiber activation during the workout. The risk of injury is also decreased.

If don't live in California or Florida, make sure to warm up properly and to wear a light sweater during the first few sets. You can still show off later.

46. What kind of cardio is best?

Basically, there are two schools of thought: old school with long duration low-intensity cardio sessions (45 to 60 minutes at a steady state) and the new school recommending high-intensity interval cardio. Who is right?

Actually, the purpose of cardio in bodybuilding is to burn off body fat and improve your cardiovascular health. The old way of doing cardio is quite effective since it keeps your heart rate at a steady level for a prolonged period of time. This is the kind of cardio I would recommend right after training with weights in order to achieve maximum fat loss. During weight training you achieve glycogen depletion, which means that the body will burn fats for energy in the follow-up cardio session.

High Intensity Interval Training (HIIT) cardio also has its merits. It creates a higher energy output than steady state cardio, and it saves time because sessions are usually only about 20 to 25 minutes. A typical session would look something like this: 8 minutes warm-up, 6 sets of 30-second sprints, 90 seconds easy, 5 minutes cool down.

Your heart rate is much higher when performing HIIT cardio and your basic metabolic rate (BMR) stays elevated for 24 hours after the session, which means you burn some additional calories after the session. If you are pressed for time, 30 minutes of HIIT will burn more calories than regular low-intensity cardio.

So why not just perform HIIT every time? Because it can be too stressful on your recovery and lead to over training. I would recommend 1 to 2 HIIT sessions on non-lifting days and 2 low-intensity sessions after your regular weight workout if maximum fat loss is your goal. Personally, I don't believe that that much cardio is warranted if your diet is in check.

47. Warming up on the treadmill works best

Warming up with cardio is another one of those things that people do without thinking because they have been told to do it. Warming up on the treadmill is a good idea if you are runner. But if you are trying to lift heavy, it's time to rethink that approach.

I am not against warming up, but you need to warm up where it is needed; that is, in your joints, which are about to bear the brunt of the labor. Someone training chest needs to warm up with light presses; ditto for back with light pulls. Leg training can be preceded by walking on the treadmill, but you need several sets of light squats on top of that to get sufficient blood flow into the knees.

You should always perform several light to medium sets of the exercise you are to perform before going into your work set. This will also put you in the proper mindset to target that muscle correctly once you start lifting heavier.

A complete warm up for better results

My idea of a warm up is more functional because most people are very unbalanced in their muscular development, and it is this that makes them susceptible to injuries. For that purpose, it is a good idea to test yourself once in a while with an overhead squat, one-legged front squat, as well as the pencil test in order to see if your flexibility and symmetry are all there.

Proper, injury-free training equals bigger muscles and less body fat. If you discover that you are indeed stiff, add some dynamic stretches, such as the wood chop, pike walk, or rotational press to your warm-up. Also, test your rotator cuff against your incline bench. You should be able to use 9% of your incline bench maximum on your cuff rotation. So, if you can bench 300 pounds, you should use 27 pounds; if you are struggling with that, an injury is coming your way.

Here's a hypothetical warm-up.

For an upper-body workout:

5 minutes light cardio
5 minutes **myofascial** work on the foam roll for lats, lower back, and sides
10 minutes weak point work such as rotator cuff and dynamic stretches, (abs work if you can't master an unanchored sit up)
2 to 4 light warm up sets of your first exercise, very controlled; focus on the squeeze and release

For the lower body workout:

5 to 10 minutes walk on treadmill

5 minutes foam roll work for hamstrings, piriformis, iliotibial (IT) bends and tensor fascia late (TFL)
5 to 10 minutes of pike walk, overhead squats and stretch lunges
2 to 3 light warm-up sets of your first exercise

A warm-up like the above will take up more time than you are used to, but it will deliver a more productive workout and keep you out of the doctor's office for longer. So overall it is a wise investment!

Part III
Diet and Nutrition

48. Grapefruits burn fat
49. Fruit is good for you
50. Exercise on an empty stomach burns more body fat
51. A calorie is a calorie
52. The body can only use 30 grams of protein per meal
53. Shakes are great for weight loss
54. I don't want to watch what I eat but rather exercise more
55. Don't eat after 6 p.m. if you want to lose weight
56. Eat only the egg whites not the yolks
57. Fats make you fat
58. The good guys among fats and why they are your friends
59. You will lose weight on a diet that calls for eating one kind of food
60. Low carbohydrate diets are best for weight loss
61. Diet sodas are good for weight loss
62. Red wine is good for you
63. Eat spinach; it contains a lot of iron
64. Salt is bad for you
65. Chocolate is bad for you
66. Asparagus has negative calories
67. I don't have to weigh my food because I can eyeball portions
68. A high protein diet can cause kidney failure
69. Granola bars are a good snack
70. There are good carbohydrates and bad carbohydrates
71. Cereal is a good breakfast
72. A cheat day a week is okay
73. Soy protein raises estrogen levels
74. As long as I eat the right macronutrients, it doesn't matter when or what I eat
75. Fatty foods go straight to the hips
76. Soup is a good diet food
77. Milk gives you thick skin
78. You should lose 2 pounds of fat a week

48. Grapefruits burn fat

Remember the Grapefruit Diet? Eat only grapefruit and lose 20 pounds in as many days. The hype surrounding this diet has dwindled, and for good reason, but the myth still lingers. Do grapefruits really burn fat? The answer is not so clear-cut.

First of all, grapefruits are truly great food. They contain a variety of antioxidants, vitamin C, and control insulin levels. Studies have shown that grapefruit aides in DNA repair, can control the growth of cancer cells in vitro, and fights Hepatitis C. This is certainly a very impressive resume overall. Yet, there is no direct correlation between the intake of grapefruit and speed of fat loss.

However, grapefruits are full of naringin, which among other things inhibits activity of the enzyme CYP34A in the human liver.

What does that have to do with fat loss? Caffeine, one of the most potent fat burners, is metabolized by CYP34A. So, the intake of naringin could lengthen the half-life and increase the activity of your fat burner therefore making it more effective. For best results you should eat the fruit with all its fiber. Grapefruit juice has shown to be less effective. A good dose would be 6 ounces of grapefruit for breakfast (no sugar!) with your thermogenic or simply black coffee.

49. Fruit is good for you

One of the first things you need to do, if you are serious about building a great physique, is to throw out the food pyramid that the U S Department of Agriculture provides. If you are going to get the majority of your calories from grains, fruit, and other sugars, you will have a better chance of becoming obese than lean and muscular. Instead of munching on bread and bagels through the day, eat 4-5 servings of lean proteins with leafy greens as well as healthy fats such as nuts, avocados, and olive oil. In addition, you can add 2 to 3 servings of complex carbohydrates a day.

So where does fruit fit into your diet? Fruit has a lot of vitamins and phytonutrients, which is great. But it also contains fructose, which is a sugar that cannot be directly absorbed, so the body sends it to the liver to be metabolized. While a small amount of fructose isn't a problem, larger quantities (more than 80 grams per day) are difficult for the body to handle. So how do you get the good stuff without too much sugar?

Stay away from fruit juices and smoothies. These things are filled with sugars and contain up to 300 grams of carbohydrates a serving. Dried fruit is a caloric nightmare, since the bulk (water) has been removed, leaving you with a high sugar item. Canned fruit is often laced with sugar and deprived of nutrients. Pick fruits that provide the most vitamins and anti-oxidants per calorie. Blueberries, grapefruit, kiwis, and strawberries are great choices.

The best time to consume fruit is with breakfast and before your workout, since fructose takes longer to digest and releases its energy over a prolonged period of time. Don't shy away from fruit altogether, but use it in moderation.

50. Exercise on an empty stomach burns more body fat

This statement actually might be true. Since the body is deprived of nutrients after not eating during the night, it will tap fat sources quicker. But there is a downside to it: in the morning, the body is inherently catabolic, which means it is beginning to strip muscle down for energy.

Working out on an empty stomach burns more muscle, which defeats the purpose of any fat loss diet. I also believe that working out in a fasting state is sub-optimal, since the lack of nutrients will not allow for peak performance.

At a bare minimum one should consume some whey protein or BCAAs in order to keep the body from using skeletal muscle for energy. Twenty to 30 grams would be an appropriate dosage. Some green tea or caffeine combined with the amino acid l-tyrosine can enhance the fat burning effect of the workout and provide a little mental edge to get on the treadmill in the morning.

If you are on a low carbohydrate diet, the timing won't make a difference since your glycogen stores will be empty at all times and conversely you will have plenty of free form fatty acids (FFA) in your blood stream.

However, one needs to keep in mind that it is overall caloric consumption over 24 hours that matters. In other words, an early workout is great but it won't be enough to off set a double cheeseburger at lunchtime!

51.   A calorie is a calorie

On the surface, yes. A calorie measures the amount of energy needed to increase the temperature of 1 liter of water by 1 cegree Celsius. But caloric balance matters. If you eat too much of any food you will gain adipose tissue (body fat).
So does it make a difference where the calories come from?

It does indeed, and there are two ways to look at it. The first is volume of food. Clean foods have more volume and are less calorie-dense than processed foods. Let's say you eat 200 grams of carbohydrates in 1 bag of Gummi Bears. To consume 200 grams of carbohydrates in clean foods, you would have to eat 6 to 7 medium baked potatoes all in one sitting. It's unlikely you'd be able to do it. It's about food volume. Clean foods have more volume; so you eat less.

Aside from food volume, there is the macronutrient breakdown: how many of your daily calories are coming from protein, fats, and carbohydrates.Consider the following: to digest 100 calories of protein, 24 to 30 calories are needed; yet, carbohydrates use only 7 calories and fats use only 3 calories. Th s is called the thermic effect of food (TEF), and it is extremely he pful when dieting. The TEF is also raised if you eat every 2 to 3 hours.

In addition, protein is a hunger suppressant and controls insulin much better than carbohydrates do. Protein also puts the body in an anabolic (muscle building) state and keeps your metabolism going. Protein comes from the Greek word *proteas*, which means "the one" or "the first". A successful diet comes down to nutrient breakdown, which is essentially the manipulation of the macronutrients according to your goals.

An appropriate nutrient breakdown—in combination with proper caloric intake—will be the difference between a person achieving nothing and a person achieving amazing results. Combined with an effective training program, there is almost ncthing a person can't achieve if they apply good science to their diet and are dedicated to the task.

The truth is that everyone is different and reacts in a different way to each macronutrient. I recommend starting with a basic 40/40/20 (40% protein/40% carbohydrates/20% fats) diet and check your results after 4 weeks. If it is not working, you might be carbohydrate sensitive and a higher protein/lower carbohydrate approach would be better for you.

Then there is satiety. In my opinion, the most successful diet is the one you can stick to. If carbohydrates help you curb your hunger best, try the Zone diet for instance. If you are like most people and consuming even a moderate amount of carbohydrates make you ravenous (I've caught myself many times rifling through the fridge at night) you will be better off with a higher protein and fat approach since your insulin levels will be more even and you won't be starving. There is also a chance that certain foods simply don't work for you, they might bloat you, make you feel sluggish (baked goods often have that effect). You will have to go through the list of foods that you consume regularly and eliminate them one by one in order to find the perfect combination for you.

Lastly, variety is key. The body becomes inefficient when it's always fed the same foods, so make sure you rotate your sources for protein, carbohydrates, and fats often.

52.   The body can only use 30 grams of protein per meal

That is one of these numbers that is frequently thrown around without much scientific backing. First off all "the body" can mean Arnold Schwarzenegger or Dakota Fanning; I highly doubt that they have the same protein requirements.

While it is a good idea to spread your protein intake throughout the day, it is also safe to assume that you can easily absorb up to 60 to 80 grams per meal if you are male and 50 grams per meal if you are female. It is not uncommon for intense trainees to consume 400 grams a day. If they broke it down to 30 grams, that would require eating 13 meals a day, which is not practical.

Another theory about protein consumption is the so-called pulse feeding plan. One study has shown that 3 big protein meals spaced out during the day and supplemented with BCAAs produced better results in terms of muscle mass gain than 6 smaller ones. The problem is that all studies regarding meal frequency are done with very few participants and none with athletes.

Whether you choose to eat 4 or 8 meals, in order to build lean mass you will need to consume 1 to 1.5 grams of protein per pound of bodyweight, along with a sufficient number of carbohydrates and fats. Depending on the size of the athlete, this should be spread out over 4 to 6 meals during the day. As for protein consumption, I'd rather err on the side of over consuming than under!

53.   Shakes are great for weight loss

There are a plethora of diet shakes flooding the market: Slim fast, Oprah's shakes, Atkins shakes, and the list goes on. Most of them contain some protein (often the cheap kind) a mix of vitamins and sugars, coloring agents, etc.

So do they work for weight loss? Not so well, I am afraid. While protein shakes are a great asset for every athlete in order to make sure there is enough protein in his diet, they don't work well for weight loss purposes. The reason is not only that the nutritional quality of most of these products is poor, but also that shakes do not satisfy your appetite for long. The vitamin mixes are unbalanced and they contain no fiber, which is the substance that will keep you satisfied and full during your diet.

Compared to foods like brown rice or chicken they take up very little stomach volume and are digested much quicker, meaning the athlete will suffer more hunger pangs. The average American consumes about 1/3 of his calories in liquid form, which is one of the reasons why the nation is facing an obesity epidemic (hello, fruit smoothie!) Liquid calories are much easier to consume than whole foods, making it harder to keep track of your actual intake.

Whole foods require more digestive work than liquids do, so they use up energy and keep the metabolism elevated. Studies have shown that test subjects consume 12 to 20% more calories when they consumed a liquid food as opposed to eating a solid meal. Their hunger responses were also worse, even the day after the liquid meal.

Whole foods also provide a wide array of phytonutrients which simply can't be duplicated as of yet. These nutrients will help to ensure optimal health and maximum fat loss. If you are very time-constricted and you simply have to use a shake, try to find some high-end whey protein and add some fats in the form of nut butters or coconut oil to it, which will increase satiety and slow down digestion. If you are on a very strict weight loss diet, just have some steamed vegetables with it—while not very tasty, the fiber will keep you full without adding considerable calories.

54.   I don't want to watch what I eat but just exercise more

Unfortunately, that doesn't work. Your diet is responsible for 70% of your appearance. There are plenty of people in the gyms who work out regularly, even possess above average strength and muscle mass but they do not have the physiques they could have because their nutritional program is off. They simply look a little bit bigger in street clothes but aren't terribly impressive on the beach. Their body fat is simply too high.

In short: you can't out-exercise a poor diet. If you do not keep your diet clean and your caloric intake within your limits you will not progress in your quest for a better body. Fat loss and muscle gain happen in the kitchen; the gym only provides the catalyst. But what if I did more cardio to offset the pizza from last night? It's not a good idea. The reasons are simple: it becomes impossible to burn off the extra calories and even if you could (one muffin requires about an hour on the treadmill to be burned), you wouldn't have consumed enough quality nutrients to build muscle.

You will need to determine your caloric needs, a sensible macro nutrient break down and stick with it. Adherence to a meal plan is the single biggest requirement to building a better physique; you will be amazed at the progress you are going to make within weeks (get ready for a lot of jealousy or compliments, depending on your environment.)

So while it is okay to indulge once in a while, you have to make sure that the vast majority of your meals are prepared toward your goals. Start by cooking your own meals to your liking and taste. This will give you a better idea about portion sizes and calorie content. Once you have gained a basic understanding of food, you will find it easier to order in restaurants without throwing your diet off.

55. Don't eat after 6 p.m. if you want to lose weight

What matters in your battle against the scale is your daily or weekly calorie consumption. So if you overeat at breakfast, you will not lose weight despite not eating after 6 p.m. But not all nutrients are created equal when it comes to their optimal time of consumption. You should eat the majority of your carbohydrates before and after your workout while protein and fats should be spread throughout the day.

One of the more esoteric diets of the last decade, the so-called warriors diet, even called for only one meal a day: dinner. People did lose weight following this protocol, but I would not recommend going 12 or more hours without food.

Since most people train after work (between 5 and 6 p.m.), it would be counterproductive not to eat after working out. After weight training, the body needs to replenish the glycogen stores as fast as possible. If this does not happen, it will use body protein (your muscle tissue) in order to fulfill its energy needs.

So after training, try to consume at least 1, better 2 meals with sufficient carbohydrate and protein content (0.5 grams of carbs and 0.3 grams of protein per pound of lean body mass would be a good proportion for this meal.) If you train in the morning, schedule most of your carbohydrates around the workout and eat mostly fats and protein at night.

Good late night snacks would be: cottage cheese with nuts, protein shake with almond butter, or small servings of meat, fish, and vegetables.

56. Eat only the egg whites not the yolks

For a long time, the bodybuilding breakfast of champions consisted of egg whites, oats, and a banana. On the surface it looks great: lean protein, complex carbohydrates, and vitamins from the fruit.

However, the egg yolk should not be left out since it is as important as the white. The yolk contains most of the vitamins and minerals in the egg, plus half the protein. Moreover, without the egg yolk, the amino acid chain is incomplete and harder to digest. Since the egg white-only breakfast is nearly fat free, it will cause a significant insulin spike and promote hunger cravings as well as energy swings later in the day. The yolk provides healthy fats, linoleic acid, and other important nutrients to control insulin release as well as additional protein.

What about cholesterol? Eggs do not contribute to someone's cholesterol balance, unless they are fried in butter and served with bacon. The fat in the yolk actually serves as a reducing agent toward LDL according to study done by the University of Connecticut. To put it in perspective, your body contains about 30 grams of cholesterol at any given time, whereas an egg yolk delivers a meager 200 milligrams. If you have high cholesterol, lower your body fat percentage before throwing out the yolk.

If you are on a very calorie restricted diet and you have little leeway in terms of calories, try to achieve at least a 2-to-1 ratio of egg whites versus whole eggs.

Lastly, there is no need to consume eggs raw. The heat from cooking them will not destroy the nutrients. If anything it will improve digestibility and get rid of any salmonella.

57.   Fats make you fat

This is one of the myths that have been around since the 80's. "Don't eat fat, it sticks to your hips. Eat our all-sugar, fat free Angel food cake instead." The results of that strategy are all around us as obesity has risen to new heights. Fats are one of the three macronutrients and are absolutely essential for good health. They absorb the vitamins A, D, E, and K, create brain and nerve tissue, regulate energy production in the mitochondria and regulate the fluids in the cell membrane.

Furthermore, fats are the building blocks for all steroidal hormones such as testosterone, estrogen, and progesterone. They also stabilize your blood glucose levels, which lead to less insulin secretion. This doesn't mean that all fats are created equal and you can have deep fried cheese for dinner. As everyone knows by now, transfats are to be avoided since they can do damage to your health.

58. The good guys among fats and why they are your friends

Essential fatty acids (EFA) are called essential because the body cannot produce those fats by itself (others can be derved from protein and carbohydrates), These EFAs are crucial to tne fat loss process because they direct mood support, lower chclesterol, reduce total triglycerides, and promote optimal focus anc concentration.

The EFAs fall into two categories: monounsaturated and polyunsaturated fats. Good sources include fatty fish, such as salmon or mackerel; nuts; avocados; and olive oil.

What does this have to do with your 6-pack abs? If you dor't consume EFAs regularly, your body will not dip into the fat deposits for energy but will instead burn muscle thereby lowering your metabolism.

In fact, to order combat the fat drought the body will store any kind of fat it can get a hold of. It will even convert protein and carbohydrates into fats in order to weather the famine. Those fats then get stored right at your love handles or belly. If your diet is too low in EFAs, you are fighting your body constantly to burn body fat.

So in order to achieve maximum fat loss you need to create a caloric deficit by increasing your expenditure and lowering your carbohydrate intake while keeping protein and essential fatty acids at sufficient levels.

Once you combine that with a well thought out weight and cardio program, all those layers will be peeled off in no time!

59. You will lose weight on a diet that calls for eating only one kind of food

The cabbage diet, the Grapefruit Diet, the cleanse, etc. These diets have been around for years and they resurge with a new magic ingredient every summer. They are at best useless and at worst dangerous. Consuming a single food over extended periods of time will lead to nutrient deficiencies and most of the weight you lose will be water and muscle since your body goes into starvation mode. During an extreme diet such as this, the body can shut down its metabolism by as much as 50% within days. After the diet is done, your body will put the weight back on since your metabolism is likely to be depressed for a while and your body fat percentage will be significantly higher than before.

Don't fall for these gimmicks; stick with one of the tried and true approaches such as high protein, medium fat, and low carbohydrates (you can still add a grapefruit if you like).

60. Low carbohydrate diets are best for weight loss

Low fat versus high fat: the diet wars are on! Just to state the obvious, any diet that causes a caloric deficit will help you to lose weight. Low fat or low carbohydrate, if you consume less energy than you burn, you will lose weight.

Let's rewind some 25 years to understand where the low carbohydrate approach comes from. During the 80's, dietary fat was the biggest villain (next to the Soviets) and was blamed for America's rapidly expanding waistline. This led to an infusion of fat-free foods such as angel food cake, Jolly Rancher, and the like. All these foods only made matters worse, the evidence of which we see all around us. So clearly, something is amiss, but what? One of the answers lies in insulin secretion, the other is simply over-consumption of carbohydrates when they are cheap and readily available.

Enter the low-carbohydrate approach, which focused on insulin control through a very restricted carbohydrate intake. The low carbohydrate/high fat diet was pioneered by (in no particular order) Dr. Seal Harries, Dr. Atkins, Mauro di Pasquale and Dan Duchaine. The approach has been constantly refined and achieved great results with thousands of users.

All this sounds great, but how do you know whether you'd get the same results? You need to find out if you gave good or bad insulin sensitivity, which means essentially: does your body handle carbs well? The test is rather simple: if you consume a high-carbohydrate meal, do you feel energized or do you crash within an hour and get sleepy and hungry?

If it's the latter, you have poor insulin sensitivity and the low-carbohydrate diet will most likely work for you. If carbohydrates make you feel energized, you would do better with a higher carbohydrate–low fat approach. The truth is that a low carbohydrate/high protein/medium fat approach has a higher success rate for most people. What constitutes a low carbohydrate diet?

Most low carbohydrate diets call for a macronutrient breakdown consisting of one gram of protein per pound of body weight and half a gram of fat. This is split over 5 to 6 high protein meals with some essential fatty acids (EFAs) and vegetables.

Most people report a steady weight loss of 2 pounds per week without a lot of cravings for junk food or hunger pangs. So all this sounds great but how does it work?

Let's look at the science. The idea is to deplete the body of glycogen (carbohydrates), which is stored in the muscles and liver, and instead use the fatty acids for energy. After 3 days of extremely low carbohydrates (the line in the sand seems to be 40 grams), the body reaches ketosis and starts burning fats instead of glucose as its primary energy source. During the state of ketosis, the body promotes fat break down, increase thermogenesis and is less likely to store fat since insulin levels are low.

Provided you create a calorie deficit through training, these fatty acids will come from your fat storage in the mid section, thighs, etc. The high protein content helps with the production of heat since the digestion of protein uses more calories than the breakdown of carbohydrates would. Furthermore, the protein helps to conserve the muscle (aided by weight training) and keep the metabolic rate from dropping. Protein is also an excellent hunger retardant, so you will have fewer late-night cravings.

Eat fats to lose fat?

It sounds counterintuitive, but during this diet, it is necessary to consume sufficient fatty acids to prevent the body from storing them. The first reaction of your body during any diet is to go into survival mode—lowering your metabolic rate and storing every calorie as fat. When provided with enough EFAs, your body will burn them off for energy since it doesn't feel deprived of them.

EFAs serve a multitude of functions in the body, but in the context of a low-carbohydrate diet they are needed as an energy source to avoid protein break down and for cell repair. They also directly assist in the fat burning process.

What role do carbohydrates play? Carbohydrates serve mainly as fuel for your body; on this particular diet the body will break down the fatty acids and use them instead of carbohydrates for energy thereby creating the weight loss. Carbohydrates are also the only one of the three macronutrients that is not essential for survival. While your brain is dependent on glucose for energy, it can create glucose from the ketones through gluconeogensis. Consuming carbohydrates also causes spikes in insulin and blood sugar. The presence of insulin makes it harder for the body to use fats for energy since it blocks lypolysis (the breakdown of fats for energy). Even on a low carbohydrate diet you will still consume some carbohydrates from leafy greens and nuts.

Every 5 to 7 days, you should have a high carbohydrate meal to keep your thyroid running and prevent your body from lowering the metabolic rate. For this meal, you can choose whatever you like. I do not recommend an all out junk fest but a nice sushi or pasta dinner instead. Make this the last meal of your day to avoid further temptations.

A Few Caveats

The problem with the low carbohydrate diet is that there is an associated water loss caused by muscle glycogen, which binds to water. With that water, you lose potassium and sodium. Sodium is usually being consumed in large enough quantities during a diet; the potassium is what presents the problem. Furthermore, the consumption of meats increases acidity in your body, which can cause joint problems. In order to combat this, you must consume alkaline vegetables with high potassium content such as asparagus, spinach, and broccoli. If you need a little bit of fruit, half a grapefruit for breakfast will also help in setting your PH-levels right. Lastly, the vegetables give more bulk to your diet and provide fiber as well as vitamins and other phytonutrients.

As for supplements, I advise taking a multi-vitamin and antioxidants during the diet. During the workout, I recommend sipping on BCAAs in order to avoid catabolism. Some people feel that this is outdated, but even if it gives you a 3% advantage, it is worth the cost.

The high success rate of the low carbohydrate diet is due to the fact that it is rather easy to follow and it produces constant results without starvation.

Here is how a typical day for a 200-pound athlete as outlined by Dave Palumbo could look like:

Meal 1:
3 to 5 whole Omega 3 eggs + 4 egg whites
1 cup of spinach
1/2 a grapefruit or blueberries

Meal 2:
50 grams whey protein
2 tablespoons of all-natural almond butter (no sugar)

Meal 3:
8 ounces chicken/halibut/turkey/tilapia
1/2 a cup cashew nuts and greens

Meal 4:
50 grams whey protein
2 tablespoons of all-natural peanut butter (no sugar added)

Meal 5:
8 ounces salmon, swordfish, or lean beef
Green salad (no tomatoes, carrots, or red peppers) with 1 tablespoon of olive oil or macadamia nut oil and vinegar

Meal 6:
50 grams whey
1 to 2 tablespoons all natural peanut butter (or almond butter) or repeat meal 1

After eating for 5 to 7 days like this, have your carbohydrate meal as the last meal of the day.

Of note: female athletes might have to include several days where they only consume lean proteins and vegetables, and every third or fourth day would be a moderate fat/high protein day as described above. The reason being that it is harder to achieve a sufficient calorie deficit otherwise.

As with any other diet, you will need to figure out your maintenance caloric levels and create a deficit from there.

Once you are satisfied with your progress you can start phasing carbohydrates back into the diet, starting with 30-50 grams on meal 1. Then add another carbohydrate meal every 7 to 10 days until you reach about one gram of carbohydrates for every pound of bodyweight.

My personal preference for staying lean is the cave man or paleo diet which includes meats, berries, leafy grains and a few grains—basically all the goodies a Neanderthal would have munched on. Some athletes have stayed on a diet like this for years with no apparent harm to their bodies; so if you do not have any underlying medical issues, give it a try.

61.   Diet sodas are good for weight loss

According to one popular diet mantra: By drinking diet soda instead of regular, you'll save tablespoons of sugar and lose weight!

This sounds great, but how much truth is there to it? While no one should consume regular sodas, diet sodas don't fare much better. Test subjects have shown an almost equal weight gain when consuming diet sodas. According to a study at the University of Texas Health Science Center, there was a 41% higher risk of being overweight for every diet soda the person drank.

But since their calorie count is undoubtly lower, how is it possible that some people still don't lose weight? There are a couple reasons for that. Studies with mice have shown that the sweeteners trigger a nearly equivalent insulin reaction as if the drinks had sugar. The insulin spike and subsequent crash leads to feeling hungry 1 hour after drinking the soda, which then can cause over-eating.

If a person is sensitive to carbohydrates, the sweet taste alone could offset the same cravings as sugar would. The person would then feel the need to consume even more carbohydrates. Also, some people may feel that they can eat more since they were so good and had a diet soda, thereby offsetting the calorie savings. I call it the diet soda/cheeseburger phenomenon.

Lastly, outside the weight loss issue there is the health concern surrounding aspartame and Splenda. Aspartame is linked to heart disease since the methanol is broken down into formaldehyde. The research is not conclusive, but it indicates that there could be a poisonous effect. While there are pro and con arguments regarding sweeteners causing cancer, I'd rather stay on the safe side and avoid them altogether.

62. Red wine is good for you

According to some people, red wine is a fountain of youth. It is full of anti-oxidants, good for the heart, prolongs your life and lowers the bad (LDL) cholesterol.

So does that mean that alcoholics turn 120 years old? Not quite. Many studies on red wine have found that the antioxidants and flavonoids, especially resveratrol, have health-enhancing effects. Resveratrol in particular is a substance of great interest. This seems to be at the bottom of the "French paradox," which is a term to describe the fact that relatively few people in France have heart problems despite a high fat diet (another reason could be the 7 weeks of vacation per year and only working 35 hours a week).

Studies with mice have shown that those that were fed a diet high in saturated fats and got a dose of resveratrol lived longer than their counterparts on a restricted diet. In fact, the resveratrol seemed to mimic the effects of a 30% calorie reduction. The substance also seems to reduce the bad cholesterol and keep the heart healthy. This and other studies have led to a surge in resveratrol supplements; it has been touted as an elixir for longevity and happiness as such. Dosages have also increased to very high levels in order to promote cell health. Now, mice are different from humans, and I am not convinced that mega dosing resveratrol is such a good idea.

So does this mean you should pound red wine to live longer?

No, for the reasons I've already explained. Because neither of these components is chemically attached to the alcohol, you can derive the same benefits from consuming grapes, grape juice, pomegranates, or a resveratrol supplement. The research on alcohol as a health inducing supplement is mixed. Some studies seem to suggest that small doses can be beneficial. A glass of red wine won't hurt you, but anything more is probably not helpful. Alcohol simply adds empty calories and causes a rise in triglycerides, which offsets the health benefits of the antioxidants, flavonoids, and resveratol.

63.   Eat spinach; it contains a lot of iron

Over the last 50 years, Popeye the sailor, who got his huge muscles from spinach, has tortured millions of kids. Here is how it all started: in 1870, a scientist named E. von Wolf published a claim that spinach contains 10 times more iron than other leafy vegetables. In 1929, Popeye was created and started wrecking havoc at dinner tables. In 1937, German scientists discovered that spinach had only 10% of the iron content that had previously been claimed. Why?

It's because, the study was done with dried spinach. In fact, the actual absorption rate of fresh spinach is even lower—somewhere in the 2 to 5% range. So since spinach does not contain a lot of iron, does that mean it is worthless for bodybuilding?

Spinach is full of antioxidants, which help fight free radicals. After a strenuous training session free radicals are released into the bloodstream to deal with the impact of the training. However, they do attack healthy cells in the body, which is why the body needs antioxidants to contain them.

More importantly, though, spinach contains beta-ecdysterone, which has shown (according to the Medicine and Science in Sports and Exercise journal) to up regulate your muscle-building abilities and speed fat loss. It is also one of the most alkaline foods you can find, which is great to offset the more acidic foods, such as meats, that a bodybuilder typically consumes in order to get your body's ph-levels more in a base range.

So in the end, your mom was right: spinach is good for you. As for iron, stick with oysters, red meat, egg yolks, and lentils.

64.   Salt is bad for you

Salt has gotten a really bad reputation. It is blamed for high blood pressure and water retention and some recommend it should be avoided altogether.

What is salt really? Salt has been around for 4,000 or more years, it was used in conserving meats and other foods. Chemically, table salt consists of two electrolytes: sodium and chloride, both of which are critical for your health. This is also the reason why you have one gustatory receptor (taste bud) just for salt. Sodium regulates blood pressure and volume; if you consume too little or too much, the body will react with changes in blood pressure. In recent years, the typical western diet has become more filled with processed foods, which are loaded with salt. This leads to an over consumption of sodium. Obese people very often eat too much sodium, which makes them reach for sugary drinks. Salty foods are also easy to eat, so calories can pile up. (Doritos?)

The real problem with sodium

The dilemma, however, is not so much the amount of sodium consumed (assuming you are watching your intake) but the potassium/sodium balance. Potassium is the counterpart of sodium in the cell, potassium gets pumped into the cell, and sodium goes out. This cycle then repeats endlessly. The potassium/sodium ratio should be around 1-to-2 but in reality it is closer to 1 to 5 since most people under-consume vegetables and overeat processed foods.

So salt itself is not the enemy, but it needs to be consumed in moderation, 2,400 milligrams a day (half a tea spoon) would be a good average. To stay on the safe side, don't eat processed foods and be careful with your saltshaker. Also make sure to consume potatoes, beans, fish, and spinach as potassium sources.

If you plan a heavy workout the next day, add a little more salt to your dinner. The extra water can help to increase your strength during the workout.

65. Chocolate is bad for you

Common wisdom has it that one of the first things that has to go in any diet are sweets, including chocolate. But it turns out there's more to chocolate than just empty calories. First, it contains high levels of serotonin, which produces a feeling of happiness. A happy dieter just might be more likely to stick to a diet.

Second, one of the fats in chocolate is stearic acid, which has some cholesterol lowering and fat burning properties. This does not mean you start packing away Snickers bars and expect to burn fat. Only very dark chocolate—70% cocoa and higher—will provide enough stearic acid. For diabetics and obese people chocolate is still off limits. If you eat it, make sure to consume only 10 grams a day due to the caloric density. As I am writing this, a Swiss company has apparently succeeded in creating a chocolate that has 80% less calories and the same taste as regular milk chocolate. It should be available in 2011, but until then you will have to keep your appetite in check.

Diets can only be successful if a person can stick to it; so if a little piece of dark chocolate helps you stay on course, by all means have it.

66.   Asparagus has negative calories

The idea that some foods require more calories to digest than they actually contain sounds great and took the diet industry by storm. It would be fantastic if there were some foods that you could actually eat and lose weight. The usual culprits are asparagus, lemon, cabbage, spinach, and apples, which were shown in one study to produce significant weight loss.

Is there any truth to it? I am afraid not. All foods have calories, and while there might be a slight calorie expenditure in digestion, it's not meaningful. Even low-calorie foods such as lettuce could cause weight gain if you consumed too much. But that is hardly possible since barely anyone could consume 6 to 8 bags of spinach per meal!

Now a diet consisting solely of spinach and lemon would not be wholesome or healthy; so it is more of an intellectual exercise than a practical possibility. Someone on this diet would probably lose a lot of weight quickly, but it would be due to malnutrition with resulting muscle loss, which would cause the drop in weight. So what about the aforementioned study? I am afraid those were patients recovering from heart surgery, not athletes in training.

Instead of speaking about negative calories, I prefer to call some foods "free foods," meaning you can eat as much as you please when dieting. These would mainly be fibrous vegetables such as asparagus, broccoli, cauliflower, cucumber, spinach, lettuce, etc. As for dressing, you can use all spices, lemon juice, and vinegar.

Any reasonable diet that is supposed to yield sustainable long-term weight loss needs to contain protein and fats (carbohydrates are optional, depending on how carbohydrate-sersitive you are). Spinach, grapefruits, and asparagus are great additions, but you simply cannot sustain yourself on them alone and expect to achieve a lean physique.

67. I don't have to weigh my food because I can eyeball portions

One of the most dangerous sentences when trying to achieve a better physique is: "I am doing pretty good with my diet." This just means the athlete has no clue how many calories he is taking in and is overeating. Studies show that people underestimate the calories they eat by 50% and they also overestimate their expenditure by about the same number. You can see where this is going. I am not saying people lie, but they are just bad at estimating calories.

I hate to be a pain here, but if you are serious about losing fat or gaining muscle, a food scale is your new best friend. After you have determined your overall caloric intake and your macro nutrient breakdown, you will have to weigh your portions. Chances are you will be surprised how easy it is to consume 100 grams of carbohydrates and on the other hand, how much food you have to eat to get 100 grams of protein (a half bag of gummi bears for the carbohydrates versus almost one pound of chicken for the protein.)

While weighing your foods sounds like a very time-consuming and tedious activity, there is light at the end of the tunnel. Most people only consume 15 to 20 foods at the most; so once you have figured out the caloric values for those foods, you will be fine. There are great Web sites such as thecaloriecounter.com or calorie-count.com that will allow you to find any food, whether it is baked, broiled, or fried within seconds. Since they can be accessed from any smart phone as well, it is possible to use them while cooking or shopping for food. Some Web sites, such as caloriecounter.com or shapeupclub.com, will even give you your daily total in a pie chart so you can compare your actual numbers against your goals.

After 3 to 4 weeks of sticking to your meals, you should be able to eat out and eyeball the portions. However, while you can estimate the size and weight, it is impossible to know how something was prepared, which can easily add up to hundreds of calories. Therefore, if you are serious about weight loss, you need to prepare the vast majority of your meals yourself.

I know that this seems very tedious and annoying but you have to understand that creating a physique is not a timely limited project but a lifetime commitment. In the end, the rewards far outweigh the sacrifices.

68. A high protein diet can cause kidney failure

The above has been used a lot to scare people out of a bodybuilding diet, but the opposite is true.

High-protein diets are usually well tolerated by healthy adults. Since your body cannot store protein, it is necessary for survival to consume it regularly. Protein is what makes your muscle, skeletal, and organ tissue as well as hair, skin, and nails. In addition, protein is responsible for your immune system and a lot of other hormonal and non-hormonal processes in the body. In short, protein is essential and not a lethal substance.

Just look at the Inuit or Eskimo people who have survived on a high-protein, high fat and very low-carbohydrate diet (not much corn grows around the North Pole) for centuries. As a result, diabetes was virtually unknown until the western-made grain products were introduced. In fact, western people didn't start farming until about 10,000 years ago; and before that they lived on meat, berries, and leafy greens.

If you are trying to gain muscle or lose fat while holding onto the muscle you have, you will need to consume more protein than a sedative person. Science has shown that a high-protein diet is not only very effective to lose weight, but it is also very helpful in keeping it off.

The question is how much is too much? I would suggest one gram of protein per pound of lean body mass. Many trainees over consume protein in the hope that more is better. But your body can only metabolize so much protein at a time; so don't go above 1.5 grams per pound of lean body mass. The higher amount would make sense during extremely strict diet phases, when the trainee is mostly eating greens and lean protein.

Unfortunately, sedentary people also tend to overconsume protein, which then comes at the cost of not eating enough vegetables and healthy fats. Without the proper enzymes and phytonutrients, the body has a difficult time digesting the protein. In many cases where people did encounter kidney or other health-related problems the cause was the overconsumption of processed, low-grade meats and the absence of vegetables as well as exercise. Many of the people who suffered side effects on a high-protein diet were also overweight and not very active. The consumption of lean, high-quality meats and vegetables has not caused health problems in the studies I have seen.

If you have an underlying or existing condition, such as kidney disease, you should check with your physician first since it might be the case that your body cannot get rid of the waste products properly.

69. Granola bars are a good snack

Granola bars are to be found everywhere these days, touted as an all-natural and healthy way of eating. Are they really?

First of all, the term all-natural can be very misleading. It has not legal definition on the United States. Natural products still have calories, and some even have a lot from sugars. Let's look at the label of one of the leading brands: 45 grams of carbohydrates, 10 grams of protein, and the primary ingredient is brown rice syrup. Yes, that is right, syrup is what holds all the nuts and oats together (cheaper brands often use high-fructose corn syrup). Any food that has a sugar derivate as its main ingredient is probably not a good choice for a physique athlete. Sometimes they use honey or agave nectar to make it healthier sounding, but it still is sugar. As a comparison: 4 ounces of Häagen Dazs strawberry ice cream have 4 grams of protein, 20 grams of carbohydrates, and 10 grams of fat and it tastes better too.

The only people who should be eating these bars, in my opinion, are extreme endurance athletes, such as cyclists or climbers in the Rockies. Because their caloric needs can be up to 10,000 a day, a high-calorie snack like a granola bar is a good addition.

If you are trying to lose fat or gain muscle, these sugar bombs should be avoided. If you really are in a pinch, eat one after your workout with some whey protein to offset the low protein content and subdue the insulin spike.

70. There are good carbohydrates and bad carbohydrates

In the age of Atkins and constantly changing diets, there is a lot of confusion about carbohydrates. Should they be avoided? Are the all bad? Which ones should I eat? It is somewhat perplexing, I admit. Think of carbohydrates as nuclear power. Used wisely, it lights up a whole city; on the other hand, it can also destroy the town (your body).

What are carbohydrates anyway? They are organic compounds consisting of ketones or aldehydes, which are linked to hydroxyl groups. In the body they are used for energy; the brain and muscles rely on glucose as a primary energy source.

Complex versus simple carbohydrates

When people refer to good and bad carbohydrates, they usually mean simple and complex carbohydrates. Simple sugars or mono- and disaccharides are sugars that have only 1 or 2 sugar molecules such as glucose, fructose, sucrose, and lactose. This means they can be digested quickly and absorbed into the bloodstream quickly. Examples include simple table sugars, dairy, jellybeans, Twizzlers, fruit, all syrups, and honey.

Complex carbohydrates are polysaccharides; they contain 3 or more sugar molecules (a potato has several hundred of these strains). They are digested more slowly and provide a longer lasting source of energy. These would be your staples such as potatoes, oats, whole-wheat pasta, bran, and brown rice.

So which ones are good and bad?

A good way to measure the impact of a carbohydrate is the glycemic index. The glycemic index or GI is a tool to measure the impact that carbohydrates have on blood sugar levels and insulin secretion. You want your blood sugars as stable as possible to avoid fat gain, fluctuating energy levels, and even diabetes.

In general, complex carbohydrates have a low GI and simple carbohydrates a high GI. There are exceptions, however.

A potato, for instance, has a GI value of 80 versus 15 for fructose. How is that possible? Fructose needs to be circulated through the liver to be digested, which causes a significant delay.

When to eat different kinds of carbohydrates

In order to achieve optimal health and a lean physique, stick with low GI foods such as yams, barley, brown rice, and whole-wheat pasta for most of your meals. There is, however, one time of the day where you want a high GI meal, and that would be right after your workout.

After working out it is critical to replenish the glycogen stores in your muscles fast and triggering the body's release of insulin can help. Insulin shuttles nutrients into the muscle cell; the faster you get those nutrients in, the quicker you can start to recover. One suggestion would be a shake consisting of whey protein mixed with a sports drink such as Gatorade or PowerAde. Other options include rice cakes with fruit preserves, white rice, white potatoes, or my all-time favorite Haribo Gummi Bears! Just make sure you consume glucose, not fructose or saccharose since these sugars won't get stored very effectively. Yes, I know what you're thinking: "is he trying to push sugar on me?" But the science is very clear on this one. Sugar is needed to cause an insulin spike, which will help to stop the muscle from wasting after working out.

I would refrain from eating carbohydrates for dinner unless you work out late. The insulin spike gets in the way of GH secretion and fat loss during the night.

Refined carbohydrates such as potato chips, sweets, cornflakes and white bread should be avoided altogether. They contain very little nutrients, and will add lots of calories to your diet.

Another way to look at carbohydrates is the way famous strength coach Charles Poliquin does; he separates them into paleo and neo carbohydrates. Paleo carbohydrates are all those a Neanderthal would have had access to such as blueberries, strawberries, and leafy greens, as well as a few grains. Neo-carbohydrates are manmade, mostly sugars and refined products. This makes for an easy separation because you automatically cut out all processed foods. The one exception would be, as mentioned above, the post-workout shake.

To sum it up: eat slow-digesting carbohydrates with your breakfast and pre-workout meal; eat fast-digesting carbohydrates right after your training session.

71. Cereal is a good breakfast

Cereal is often touted as natural and healthy when in reality it is neither. First of all, the nutritional profile is off. They contain mainly carbohydrates, very little protein, and often a random mix of vitamins. Some brands contain up to 20 grams of sugar per serving (you are likely to eat 2 servings in one sitting) some of them coming from high-fructose corn syrup.
And while the better cereals contain mostly whole grains and even deliver some fiber, there is still a lack of protein content and the fact that they are processed foods.
You will do yourself and your physique a favor by making your own breakfast. If you are bored of egg whites and oats, here is an alternative:

1 scoop of vanilla whey
3/4 cup of instant oatmeal (the perfect food)
1 cup apple (or pear) diced
1 tablespoon of natural almond butter
Cinnamon
Mix the whey and oats, add water and cook in microwave for 1 to 1.5 minutes. Add in apple and almond butter, sprinkle with cinnamon.

There you have it: high protein, complex carbohydrates, and healthy fats. This breakfast should satisfy your hunger as well as your taste buds.
If you are on a low-carbohydrate diet, I would recommend a spinach omelet with some grilled chicken breast (or lean beef). I use low-fat cheese to give it more taste.

72. A cheat day a week is okay

Most diets these days allow for some sort of cheat meal or cheat day during the week. This makes sense because it enables the athlete to stick with the plan since there is light at the end of the tunnel, and it prevents the metabolism from dropping.

It a so comes in handy if you have to attend a social event like a wedding or birthday party.

The question is: what is a cheat day, how much of a cheat meal/day is needed, and can a cheat day be counterproductive? A cheat day can mean two things: carte blanche (eat what you want) or have one meal to your liking while the remaining meals are still within the diet plan.

The answer depends on how much of a calorie deficit is the athlete in and what kind of diet is he following. Let's cover the deficit aspect first. If someone goes into a really deep deficit (cutting calorie intake by 50%) while still training hard, a cheat day would actually be needed.

Why a cheat day makes sense

So you are dieting, cutting your calories, upping the cardio, etc. You are all set for a gradual fat loss of 1 to 2 pounds per week. After all, you did the math and created a calorie deficit.

Unfortunately, your body hates you. Actually it loves you so much that it wants to keep you alive and prevent death by starvation. So it makes some adjustments, which were great for the hunters and gatherers but bad for a physique athlete.

What are those adjustments?

After a couple days of dieting, the metabolism slows down, hunger increases, and more and more muscle mass is sacrificed by the body for energy. The human body is very efficient at adapting to new conditions.

In short, thyroid hormone T3 levels drop by 30%; conversion from T4 to T3 in the liver is being slowed down, the half-life of cortisol increases and the production of Insulin like growth factor (IGF-1) is down.

Your muscles are so low on glycogen that they are resistant to growth despite training. Leptin, a messenger hormone, is an important player in the diet scenario because it normally inhibits your appetite to prevent you from overeating and gaining weight.

Now when you are dieting, the opposite holds true. With the reduced calories, leptin levels drop and appetite goes up. This means that a person who lowers his body fat is at an immediate disadvantage: His metabolism is automatically slowed down by as much as 20% within days.

So during a diet, all of a bodybuilder's nightmares come together: higher protein turnover combined with a lower levels of T3, IGF-1 (insulin like growth factor, one of the strongest muscle building hormones), leptin, and testosterone. All this happens despite training and after only several days, not months, of dieting. Very soon the athlete reaches a plateau; no fat is lost and instead lean body mass is sacrificed.

Can this be stopped?

Yes, in some cases people simply use drugs. Testosterone, human growth hormone, and insulin are injected, combined with oral thyroid medication. For a natural bodybuilder this is not an option. We need to find a way to manipulate the body's hormones for a short time.

This can be achieved with a refeed. In order to prevent the above-mentioned adaptations, it is necessary to increase the calories and to refeed every 5 to 7 days. A refeed is basically an intelligent cheat day where calories are increased from 130% to 150% of maintenance. Increasing the calories for a short period of time reverses the process described above. Testosterone, IGF-1, and leptin levels are brought up; the production of cortisol is slowed down; as a result, the rate of metabolism increases, which then sets the stage for further fat loss.

How to do a proper refeed

The calories during a refeed should come mainly from carbohydrates, moderate protein, and very low fats. I recommend 4 to 5 grams of carbohydrates per pound of bodyweight over a 24-hour period with about one gram of protein per pound of body mass and trace fats (i.e., only what's in food). So a 200-pound athlete would be eating 800 to 1,000 grams of carbohydrates and 200 grams of protein.

Why should I eat carbohydrates? Won't I get fat by eating so much?

You will not. Adding carbohydrates to a diet at this particular point, as opposed to protein or fats, has several advantages. Leptin, insulin, and blood sugar levels are being up-regulated, but due to the temporary lack of enzymes, the body is unable to store body fat. The body's first order of business is to refill glycogen storage, which takes about 24 hours; after that fat storage starts. Imagine someone with a $10,000 credit card balance with 24% interest. If this person gets $10,000 he will pay off the credit card, not start a savings account. The credit card balance is your muscle glycogen; the savings account your fat cells. Too bad this awesome window is only open 24 hours.

A cheat day or refeed can be made more effective if the dieter does a heavy workout after his carbohydrate day. This ensures the glycogen gets taken into the muscle. The refeed day would be an ideal time to work on a weaker muscle group and use the insulin response for new growth.

So, let me sum up how I would structure a diet and training program for an already lean athlete.

Monday:
Very low carbohydrates high fat/medium protein
45 minutes of weight training, focus lower body,

Tuesday:
Repeat diet
Train upper body

Wednesday:
Same diet
Cardio if needed, no weights

Thursday:
Whole body workout
Start carbohydrate up right after workout

Friday:
No training
Refeed. The rule of thumb would be 16 grams of carbohydrates for every kilogram of lean body mass within a 36-hour period

Saturday:
Train lagging muscles heavy
Eat a regular Zone diet

Sunday:
Back to Monday's diet
Cardio if needed

Now what about someone with a more moderate calorie deficit?

The body's hormonal response during the diet is similar to that of an extreme calorie deficit. Cortisol will be elevated, testosterone suppressed, and the metabolism slowed down. However, since glycogen stores are probably not completely empty, I suggest only a single high-carbohydrate cheat meal to avoid the possibility of fat storage. Depending on the size of the athlete, 200 to 500 grams of carbohydrates should be sufficient in order to replenish glycogen and speed up the thyroid. Varying caloric intake every few days is a great way to keep your metabolism running. A popular way of doing it would be a 2 days low, 1 day high carbohydrate scheme like this:

Monday:
Moderate caloric deficit (300-500 calories), 100 to 150 grams of carbohydrates, regular weight training
Tuesday:
Repeat
Wednesday:
Consume twice the amount of carbohydrates, lower your fats, no weight training
Thursday:
Back to Monday's diet, work on weak body part
If you don't feel fuller by Thursday, you might have to do a 2 days high/2 days low diet.
I don't believe in all-out junk fests. Even on a cheat meal you should consume mostly clean foods and maybe have a small dessert or a side of fries with your steak. So the cheat meal is not a myth; it is a necessity if you diet correctly. For anyone who has further interest in this topic, I highly recommend *Bodyopus* by Dan Duchaine and *The Ultimate Diet 2.0* by Lyle McDonald.

73. Soy protein raises estrogen levels

Soy protein has fallen in and out of favor in the bodybuilding community in recent years, which is a shame because it is a very valuable protein. Its biological value is not that high (74), but it seems to have some cholesterol lowering properties. It is a great choice for lactose-intolerant athletes as well as vegetarians.

The whole estrogen question is a bit sketchy since there are conflicting studies, and the findings differ between men and women. I will try to give both sides of the argument. Soy does contain pythoestrogens, which can affect estrogen levels in the body by docking on to the estrogen receptor and sending a weak signal to produce estrogen. For most women, slightly higher estrogen levels would most likely not be a huge deal. This is likely why most studies done on women have not produced any conclusive findings.

Needless to say, men should try to stay away from elevated estrogen levels. But the question is: does soy really increase those levels to a degree where performance could be harmed?

One would have to consume a large amount of soy over a long period of time. The studies I have read differ in their findings but no study reported enough of a drop in testosterone to inhibit performance. Since soy users have reported muscle growth, I have a hard time imagining that this could have happened on low testosterone levels.

I would, however, limit my soy intake to 25 grams after the workout with 25 grams of whey. That should be enough to reap the antioxidant benefits of the soy.

Soy protein is often used in protein bars and cereal, so if you consume a lot of these products, you wouldn't need a soy concentrate. As for a particular product, I would recommend soy isolate since it has been cleaned of carbohydrates and fats and will be digested quicker.

74. As long as I eat the right macronutrients, it doesn't matter when or what else I eat.

This is a 2-for-1 myth; so I will tackle them in order. Yes, macronutrients are critical. Without a proper balance of proteins, carbohydrates, and fats there won't be any change in your body. So can you just eat any foods, as long as the carbohydrate/protein/fats ratio is okay?

No, sorry, the particulars do matter—not all foods and all people are created equally. Certain foods will work better with your body than others. If you have ever tried to get all your protein from solid food sources as opposed to shakes, you will probably have noticed that you are fuller and more muscular when consuming more chicken and fish as opposed to protein powder.

The same goes for carbohydrates. Some people can handle oats very well while others get stomach discomfort and a bloated look. These things matter tremendously in your appearance; you will need to find out which ones are right for you. In my case, red meat works very well for me when I am stressed out and rundown and chicken just doesn't cut it.

When to eat what or nutrient timing

Proper nutrient timing can make or break your entire program.

Here are my nutrient timing rules:
1. Every meal needs to contain protein in order to keep a steady pool of amino acids in the blood stream.
2. Carbohydrates are not a meal; they should not be eaten alone. Eating carbohydrates by themselves will cause an insulin spike and a crash later on, which will facilitate fat storage.
3. Split your carbohydrates evenly between breakfasts and pre- and post-workout meals. If you take in 50 grams of carbohydrates a day, split it 50/50/50. By doing this you will provide sufficient energy for the workout as well as speeding up the recovery afterwards. The post-workout meal is crucial. Not only will it speed up rebuilding but you will also actually burn more calories than eating nothing because it keeps the metabolism high. I recommend a liquid meal such as Gatorade and whey protein as this will get into your blood steam quicker than solid foods.
4. No carbohydrates for dinner unless it is your post-workout meal. When you eat carbohydrates late in the day, they interfere with the growth hormone release, which is your best natural fat burner. Good dinner choices include steak and leafy greens, salmon and asparagus, or chicken with greens and cashews.
5. Try to eat as little fat as possible in the pre- and post-workout meal since it will slow down digestion.

6. Try to eat at least 5 to 6 meals. Cramming all your nutrients into 3 meals will not make for a better physique. Insulin swings are going to be too big and your body will not be anabolic enough to build mass and lose fat. Two of those meals can be shakes; the rest should come from solid food sources.
7. Most importantly: *Do not miss meals.* If you really want to improve your physique, then you can't miss meals for weeks or even months. If you are in training and you miss a meal, your body will use protein (muscle mass) for energy and will be more inclined to store fat the next time you eat. You will need to plan your days ahead of time, especially if you travel. Sorry, but there are no shortcuts.

If you can stick to these 7 guidelines, you will notice a tremendous difference in your energy levels as well as performance.

75. Fatty foods go straight to the hips

The myth is that when you consume heavy foods, they are stored directly in the fatty deposit areas like the thighs and hips. Really?

This needs to be broken down by sex since men and women's bodies handle fat storage differently. Men tend to have less body fat and store more of it as visceral fat (a beer gut). Men also have more fatty acids floating in the blood stream, which makes it easier for guys to lose weight, but also makes them more susceptible to a heart attack. Women store the majority of fat in the hips and thigh area, which was intended by nature to secure the survival of our species. Women can survive longer in a time of famine because they carry more fat on their bodies.

So what happens after the last slice of pie is wolfed down at Thanksgiving dinner? Studies conducted after a heavy meal (100 grams of fat or the equivalent of a double cheeseburger with fries) as well after a carbohydrate heavy meal show that blood flow to fat cells doubles. Women experienced increased blood flow in the thigh and hip region, where they tend to accumulate fat; whereas men experienced a broader increase in blood flow because they tend to store fat throughout the body. In either case, it is a very good argument against over-eating in one sitting. So your mom was right after all.

Try to space your meals out over the day and keep carbohydrates to about 30 to 50 grams per sitting. The one exception would be after training where you can consume up to one gram per pound on lean body mass.

Overconsuming calories, regardless of which kind, leads to increased fat storage, wild energy swings and crashes as well as trouble concentrating.

Try to avoid it!

76.   Soup is a good diet food

Soups are being sold as a healthy low-calorie food and are a very convenient lunch. But what is their value for an athlete?

I hate to be the bad news guy again, but most packaged soups have no place in an athlete's diet. They usually contain up to 2,000 milligrams of sodium per serving (your daily allowance), are heavy in carbohydrates, and low in protein. In addition, most commercial soups deliver 4 to 5 grams of saturated fats per serving. Since some of them are sold with crackers, the carbohydrate content is even higher without any real nutritional value.

There are times when soups can he helpful. During a strict diet bouillon can work wonders to curb hunger. At a social event ordering minestrone soup to start the meal will fill you up and save you a lot of calories later on.

Other than that, steer clear of soups unless you make them yourself.

77.   Milk gives you thick skin

For a long time it was believed that milk made you smooth, obscuring your precious muscularity. This comes from two different, entirely unrelated, reasons. First, before the advent of protein powders, bodybuilders used to bulk up on copious amounts of milk and cream, often a gallon or more per day. That kind of a caloric intake would leave anyone smooth. Second, milk and dairy products contain sodium, which can cause water retention under the skin. However, this is only a problem for folks who are already very lean. An obese person is not going to look better or worse because of water retention.

So should dairy products be banned from a diet? That depends on several factors. If you are on a very strict ketogenic diet, the lactose content of most products might cause problems. For the vast majority of all other dieters, cottage cheese, or low fat Greek yogurt can be a good addition. For once, the casein in those products digests slowly, so it suppresses hunger quite well. Dairy also delivers calcium, which then binds ingested dietary fats so it can help with shedding some pounds.

As with any food, this is all very individual, you simply have to try it and see if it works for you.

78.   You should lose 2 pounds of fat a week

This section should be called "why the traditional approach to dieting is flawed." The above is a standard recommendation by many people in the industry and that is exactly the problem. It is too generic a statement and will not work for most people. Larger individuals can lose more than 2 pounds per week whereas smaller athletes might be only able to lose a half a pound per week. It is a simple matter of science. A pound of fat contains about 3,500 calories. That's 7,000 calories for 2 pounds. In order to lose that in a week, the daily deficit would have to be 1,000 calories, if you were to burn only fat, which is a poor assumption in the first place as the body never uses fat exclusively as a source of energy.

As an example, a small female athlete with a BMR of only 1,300 calories would have to add 2 hours of cardio a day to achieve that kind of a deficit, which is simply not practical.

On the other hand, a large male who has a maintenance requirement of 3,500 calories can easily diet on 2,000 calories a day with proper refeeds and training in order to drop body fat somewhere in the range of 3 pounds a week.

So how is it that smaller dieters sometimes drop larger amounts of weight rather fast? Because they are losing body weight not necessarily fat, but more likely muscle. Since they are underfed and overtrained, these dieters are burning through their muscle at a rapid rate. This will make them smaller but not leaner.

How is this possible? Since muscle is all protein, a pound of muscle yields only 600 calories. So even somebody with a smaller deficit can lose a lot of "weight" if that person overtrains.

An ideal diet has to try to maintain muscle mass while keeping performance at a high level. *The Ultimate Diet 2.0* by Lyle McDonald is a fantastic read if you have further interest. In the meantime, here are my 10 diet commandments:

1. Calories matter! You can't expect to lose weight by just manipulating macronutrients. Whatever diet you choose (low-carbohydrate, low-fat), you need a deficit. 80% of that deficit should come from your diet, the rest from exercise.

Contrary to popular belief, you need to exercise less while dieting since your recovery is impaired due to the lack of nutrients (this only applies to active people).

If you train more and eat less, you will lose muscle and look worse than before.

Don't go below 1,000 calories a day. If you are a smaller dieter, you need to add aerobics to create a sufficient deficit and set yourself up for a longer diet.

2. Eat 1.5 grams of protein per pound of lean body weight. If your performance drops, up that amount to 2 grams per pound. Women should be fine with 1 to 1.5 grams.

3. Add 10 grams of fish oil to your diet as well as a multivitamin. Eat several servings of fibrous vegetables a day for fullness. Asparagus, eggplant, spinach, cauliflower, broccoli, lettuce, and celery can be eaten in unlimited quantities.

4. Train with weights at least 2 to 3 times a week for 45 to 50 minutes, try to hit every muscle twice a week.

5. Drop your volume in the weight room, not your intensity. You need to cut back on sets but not on weight on the bar. Overall volume can be dropped by (gasp) two-thirds, so if you were doing 6 heavy sets for your chest, you would end up with 2. This will significantly reduce the time you spend in the weight room and allow you to recover on reduced calories.

6. Do not start doing cardio every day as you will over train and burn through muscle.

7. Plan refeeds accordingly depending on body fat level. Here is a breakdown:

Re-feed frequency according to body fat levels

Men	Less than 10% body fat	10-20% body fat	More than 20% body fat
Re-feed every	5 days	10 days	2 weeks
Women	Less than 20% body fat	20-30% body fat	More than 30% body fat
Re-feed every	S7 days	10 days	2 weeks

8. If your performance in the weight rooms drops significantly (more than 10%), you must up your calories by 10 to 15% in order to avoid muscle loss. Most of those calories should come from protein.

9. Stay alert for loss of appetite, elevated pulse, and irritability. Those are signs of overtraining and you will have to break the diet when they occur. Otherwise, you will lose a great deal of muscle, which will leave you looking much worse than before you started your diet.

10. Plan your cheat and refeeds properly so you can have a life. Strict dieters are more likely to fail in their quest than people who leave room for social events. Just get back on the wagon the next day.

Contrary to many books on the subject, dieting is work and I will not give you a magic bullet (if I had one I'd be retired!) But if you follow the above guidelines, you will drop fat quicker than you think while maintaining muscle.

A lot of people gravitate from diet to diet and fat burner to training system, only to realize later that they should have just dropped calories.

Save yourself the detour and get ripped now!

Part IV
Supplements

79. I'd look a lot better if I took steroids
80. Steroid replacements are just as good as steroids
81. The 5 best supplements are…
82. Fat burners will get me lean
83. Creatine is bad for the kidneys
84. I don't need a multivitamin
85. Cellulite creams help to tone the "problem areas"
86. Diuretics or water tablets will help you get lean
87. Green tea burns fat
88. Sports drinks are necessary during a workout
89. Protein bars are good for you
90. Energy drinks before a workout give you an edge

79. I'd look a lot better if I took steroids

No book on training would be complete without mentioning steroids. While the topic is highly controversial, I feel it is necessary to address it because it is one of the most misunderstood matters in the world of fitness.

While steroids are without a doubt powerful and make a difference in athletic performance and muscle mass, they are not miracle pills. Steroids are hormones, namely testosterone, estrogen, progesterone, and cortisol. For performance-enhancing purposes, anabolic steroids are used; those are either synthetic testosterone or testosterone derivatives.

So do they work? Yes, they work very well; there is no question about it. Anabolic steroids allow the athlete to build muscle and lose fat faster. (They are also illegal in the U.S. and their possession is a felony). They aid in recovery, making it possible for the athlete to train harder and more often.

But consider this: There are an estimated several million steroid users in the US, but not all of them have amazing physiques.

Building a physique is not just about heaping on muscle or being super ripped. Quite a number of people have ruined their physiques with excessive steroid use, which can result in a bloated midsection, water retention, or acne. A 20-inch arm on a 40-inch waist does not look nearly as good as an 18-inch arm on a 32-inch waist.

More mass at any cost does not make a champion. Steroids also have side effects that can be very harmful to your health. In my opinion, bodybuilders looked a lot better in the 70's with small waists and broad shoulders than with the bloated guts you see onstage today.

As for pro athletes from other sports, they have reached their limits after years and years of training and are now looking to improve upon their already extremely high performance level. They tend to react better than most people to steroids, but it is not the drugs that make them who they are. Athletes at that level have a better bone structure and a higher percentage of fast-twitch fibers than average trainees. Most importantly, though, pro athletes are incredibly committed to their craft. No drug on the planet can replace a proper training and nutritional program, which is where most people fail in the first place. Food is, by far, the most anabolic substance on the planet (along with water).

The key component to success in building a physique is consistency, which means no missed meals or missed workouts over a period of several months or years.

Those who make it to the pro level do not owe their success to some miracle drug but to his or her commitment to diet and training. Bodybuilding is one of the few sports that requires 24/7 devotion. Most people reach for steroids long before they have fulfilled their natural potential, thereby cutting short their natural potential. You will have to find a routine that works for you; stick to your diet day in and day out, and most importantly, stay motivated!

80.   Steroid replacements are just as good as steroids

Nothing, absolutely nothing works like steroids. Steroids are prescription drugs and illegal in this country as well as banned by all major sports organizations. These powerful medications are responsible for the freakish developments you see on the pro level in any sport. Companies selling steroid replacements will pose it this way: why risk a felony charge and harmful side effects when steroid replacements will do the trick for $29.99? It is certainly a great marketing ploy, but it's just not true. Steroid replacements will not give the same results as a cycle of steroids would.

Most steroid replacements are a mix of herbal substances with little, if any, research behind them. I'm sorry, but in terms of effectiveness eggplant extract just can't beat testosterone and growth hormone. You would be better off spending $60 on steak and potatoes in order to grow muscle mass.

In order to achieve your goals, you will need to create a lifestyle that enables you to stick with your training, diet, and recovery. These 3 pieces are 90% of success; and yet, this is where most people fail. This is also why the supplement industry sells billions of dollars worth of dreams every year.

Supplements have become a lot more effective over the last decade. Things like creatine, glutamine, and whey protein can certainly help you to achieve your goals but they are not as powerful as the illegal drugs.

Just remember that they are called supplements because they are supposed to add to an already sound training and nutritional regimen. Adding a protein shake with creatine to a diet high in fast food will not make you look any better.

81. The 5 best supplements are…

So here goes in no particular order: whey protein, creatine, green foods, glucosamine/chondroitin, and fish oil.

Whey

Whey should be a staple in everyone's stack. It is the protein derived from cow's milk, fat- and carbohydrate-free (in many cases also cleaned of lactose) with the highest bioavailability, meaning your body can easily use it to create muscle mass. Whey contains all essential amino acids; so it is a complete protein with a heavy dose of BCAAs (branched chain amino acids). These amino acids have been shown to stop muscle loss after training and speed up the recovery process. Whey protein helps with fat loss since it has a thermic effect, which means it causes the body to use more energy during the digestive process. Whey causes the release of two appetite-suppressing hormones: cholecystokinin (CCK) and glucagon-like peptide-one (GLP-one), which is a godsend for anyone dieting.
It also strengthens your immune system since it is rich in the amino acid, cystine, and stabilizes your blood sugar levels.
These are the reasons whey is the number 1 selling supplement. There are many good brands to choose from: a good way to test if a particular whey protein is right for you is to take it in the morning on an empty stomach. If your alertness spikes within 30 minutes, you have a winner.

Fish oil

Fish oil capsules are an invaluable addition to any diet. The typical western diet is too low in EPA/DHA fatty acids and fatty fish or fish oils provide those nutrients. These fatty acids help with energy production and fat loss as well as supporting your memory and cognitive abilities. Most importantly, they aid in cell repair, which leads to a quicker recovery after workouts. I recommend 6 to 10 grams daily.

Green foods

Green foods or super foods are basically dried and pulverized vegetables and fruits. Nobody eats the recommended 5 to 7 servings of fruits and vegetables a day, and even if you did, you couldn't be sure to get all the nutrients you needed. With one scoop of the powder a day, green foods are a cheap and easy way to cover your needs without getting an extra serving of fructose. Taste wise, these supplements have come a long way; so while I still would not call them gourmet food, they are certainly tolerable. They also come in very handy while traveling.

Creatine

Creatine is one of the very few proven muscle-building supplements out there. With years of research and countless studies behind it, it can be deemed safe and effective. Creatine is a naturally occurring substance, found in red meat or fish—essentially 3 amino acids bonded together. The name Creatine is derived from the Greek word Kreas, which means flesh. In our bodies most creatine is stored in the skeletal muscle.

Simply speaking, creatine (phosphocreatine) increases muscle energy availability. The cells of our body store their energy in the form of a molecule known as Adenosine –Tri-Phosphate, or ATP. The amount of work our muscles can perform is a direct consequence of the amount of ATP they have stored as well as the ease with which ATP is regenerated with the help of PCr (polymerase chain reaction) during anaerobic exercise.

Think of ATP as the cell's energy spending money and phosphocreatine as a debit card with an adjustable balance—the balance set by creatine deposit via the diet. Creatine tends to work best for activities that require a high strength output and last 50 seconds, which is pretty much your typical training set.

In terms of your training your muscles will be able to perform longer, at a higher output, and recover more quickly. It is not uncommon for trainees to report a 5 to 10% strength gain in basic exercises when using creatine.

Strength gain and the ability to perform at a higher level for a longer period of time leads to an increase in skeletal muscle mass. Creatine also enhances recovery, which allows you to train harder and more often. It allows the muscle cells to absorb water, meaning you will grow while using creatine. This water weight will be lost once you stop taking creatine but the added bulk while you're taking it makes for a good motivator. As for dosage, 5 grams a day is sufficient for most athletes. For beginners, I would recommend training 12 to 18 months without using creatine, because you won't reap the full benefits if you use it too early. You should have a good mind/muscle connection established before using supplements so that you can actually take advantage of the ability to train harder and heavier. Five grams a day would be sufficient; the often-proposed loading phase is, in my opinion, not necessary.

Glucosamine and chondroitin

Glucosamine and chondroitin are important to preserve joint health. Lifting weights can be harsh on your joints and ligaments; these two substances provide the building blocks for your body to replenish these areas, which can also be helpful in mitigating arthritis.

Glucosamine is made from the shells of shellfish, lobsters, or other sea creatures and is used to replenish the body's own glucosamine stores. Since the production of glucosamine slows with age, it would be wise to supplement.

Chondroitin is naturally present in cartilage and gives the ligaments elasticity and it is believed to stop the destruction of ligaments by enzymes. Since most of us don't eat cartilage or ligaments, supplementation makes sense.This is a supplement that you should use for general health and as a preventive measure. 1,500 milligrams a day would be appropriate.

These are the 5 top supplements I would recommend (glutamine is a close number 6); as staples of everyone's stack. They are tried and true, backed up by real science. Before you waste your hard-earned money on new supplements with outrageous claims, try these in combination with a proper diet and training program. You won't be disappointed—just don't expect to gain 25 pounds of muscle mass in 10 days.

82. Fat burners will get me lean

For the most part fat burners contain caffeine and or green tea, B-vitamins and yohimbine or taurine. While these substances all have some merit, they are not miracle drugs.

Fat burners do raise your metabolic burn rate, but it is only by 4 to 5%, which for a person who needs 2,000 calories a day would be 80 to 100 calories. So, if your diet is off by 500 or more calories, it won't make a difference. In comparison, a glass of wine is about 120 calories and a muffin can set you back up to 500.

The main benefit of any fat loss product lays not so much in the actual fat burning but in the hunger suppression and the added energy they provide. That extra edge (mainly coming from the stimulatory effects of caffeine) helps the calorie-deprived athlete to push through his workouts, even when hungry and fatigued. Trust me, if you are really dieting, a serving of caffeine can be a godsend for your mood and energy levels.

Caffeine also helps to burn off more free fatty acids in your blood stream while you're exercising. Yohimbine can be helpful (up to a point) in up-regulating norephedrine, which causes greater thermogenesis (heat production) and lypolysis (break down of fatty tissue). Some people might experience nausea from taking yohimbe; for those, a topical application seems more promising. Other substances that can be helpful include green tea, l-tyrosine, and synephrine.

However, when starting a diet, you need to determine your caloric needs precisely, create a deficit, and follow a reasonable exercise program. The Benedict Harris formula is particularly useful for this (http://www.bmi-calculator.net/bmr-calculator).

Try to avoid going too deeply into a calorie deficit because your body is more likely to use muscle for fuel when faced with an extreme situation. A reasonable goal is to lose 1 to 2 pounds per week; anything more and you are most likely sacrificing muscle mass. Larger athletes (over 200 lbs) can lose more than that; but you've got to keep an eye on your performance in the weight room. If your performance is dropping by 10 to 15%, you need to increase your calories by 10%.

I find it critical to have a log, maybe two: one for your meals and the other for your workouts. Write down how you felt during your workout and mark down your energy levels. Be precise in terms of your goals.

A good way to approach a cutting phase is to start changing your food intake and then, after 3 to 4 weeks, add in some low-intensity cardio. Once your diet progress slows, it can be helpful to incorporate a fat burner to make further inroads and mobilize those last stubborn fat cells. If you start cardio and fat burners too early, there is a chance you will over-train and end up sacrificing muscle.

While a fat burner can provide the extra 5 to 7%, it is crucial to get the other 95% first. They can be helpful but don't depend solely on them for your success.

A note of caution: If you are considering using DNP, which is an illegal medication, I urge you not to. While DNP can be very effective, it has caused several fatalities from stroke and being cooked from the inside. Do not use this product!

83.   Creatine is bad for the kidneys

There isn't any medical proof that a healthy, well-hydrated trainee could not tolerate the exogenous creatine. Creatine is a natural substance and can be found in red meat. It improves the body's ATP response and pulls more water into the muscle cell, which is why you need to drink more. The athlete usually experiences a couple pounds of weight gain and a 5 to 10% strength increase. The strength gains create a psychological advantage which leads to more intense training and greater gains overall.

In addition, creatine improves recovery ability so that the athlete can train harder and more often. Creatine is one of the few proven and valuable supplements. Hundreds of studies have confirmed its safety and effectiveness. In addition to its proven muscle-building abilities, studies (although with mice) even suggest an anti-aging effect.

Unless you have a pre-existing kidney condition, you should be fine using this product. Keep the dosages around 5 grams a day and take a break every 8 weeks just to be safe. You could combine that break with a week off from training to allow your body to recover fully.

84. I don't need a multivitamin

No matter how hard you try, it is nearly impossible to consume all necessary vitamins through food (is there anyone out there who consumes 8 servings of fruit and vegetables a day?)

It comes down to stomach volume. Vegetables just take up too much space and are sometimes not practical in daily life. Fruit juices do deliver the vitamins but also a lot of fructose which adds up to extra calories. And even if you managed to eat all your vegetables, you could not be sure that you were getting the nutrients. Modern agriculture has depleted our soil to such an extent that it is very difficult to accurately measure the nutrients in, say, a carrot. This doesn't mean you should solely depend on a multivitamin, but it could be a useful daily addition. Multivitamins have come a long way. Today the absorption rate of synthetic vitamins is much higher and there are many good brands out there.

But even the best multivitamin does not deliver all the nutrients you need. There are about 80 phytonutrients in an apple that we are not able to categorize yet. Furthermore the ratio of nutrients is arbitrarily adjusted so it can never be exactly right for a given individual.

For those of you who prefer to rely on Mother Nature, which I recommend, go with a green drink powder, essentially dried vegetables and fruits. This is an easy way to get 8 servings a day without having to consume the volume of food that 8 salads would deliver. Even then, I would try to eat several portions of vegetables a day for their fiber content. This becomes especially important when dieting, because the fiber will keep you from getting hungry.

85. Cellulite creams help to tone the problem areas

This section could be titled "Stubborn fat deposits and how to fight them," but I decided to go with cellulite creams since that is what most women are concerned with (for men it would be the lower abdominals and lower back area). Back to the rubs/creams: A lot of women have tried them. The ads for them are plentiful and promising and their prices range from 20 to 120 dollars. They promise firm skin by getting rid of unattractive dimples and orange skin.

Do they work? To answer that, we'll need to understand the science behind them. Cellulite is the buildup of unsightly fat cells and toxins underneath the skin, often encouraged by hormonal changes in a women's body, a genetic predisposition, prolonged periods of sitting and a poor lifestyle.

Your first line of defense when it comes to cellulite should be diet and exercise. You should work the surrounding muscles: the gluteus, hamstrings, and quadriceps. Exercises like stiff legged dead lifts, squats, and walking lunges (these are particularly effective) will target those muscle groups. Walking on a steep incline (15%) would be another way to target those areas. The better trained those muscle groups are, the more likely it is that (in combination with a proper nutritional program) the surrounding fat cells will shrink.

But let's assume you have done all the above and you still can't get rid of those last stubborn fat cells. You've added more cardio to your training, watched your diet, and, still, you are carrying these nasty little buggers.

How does fat loss occur? (Warning: more science coming up but well worth reading.)

It is generally accepted that fat loss is stimulated by the sympathetic nervous system (SNS) which sends out epinephrine and nor epinephrine. They are mainly released during flight or fight situations but your body is constantly producing them. These "messenger" substances fulfill a variety of processes in the body, but for now we only look at how they are connected with fat loss.

Fat cells don't get much blood circulation so we have Alpha and Beta adrenoreceptors for these two hormones in the fat cell. Beta-receptors are great; they initiate lipase, the enzyme that starts to break down fats into energy. The fat then becomes free fatty acids and glycerol and is used for energy. This process works only if there is no insulin present, so a low carbohydrate diet is advisable in order to keep insulin levels low.

Alpha-2 receptors are evil: they block the release of lipase and decrease the amount or nor epinephrine. These receptors sit mainly at—you might have guessed—your buttocks and love handles. And it gets worse: if you continue to diet and do excessive cardio, the number of Alpha-2 receptors will rise and you end up losing muscle along with very little fat from this problem zone.

African tree bark to the rescue?

It is possible to block the Alpha receptors with yohimbe. Yohimbe is an African tree bark, used for male potency. It is also an Alpha-receptors antagonist, but it's most effective as a topical cream and is not very effective when taken orally. A topical cream with yohimbe, aminophylline (a vasilodator for the blood vessels) and caffeine will have an effect on someone who is already lean. Studies have shown measurable improvements after a 4-week application.

If you combine the cream with a low carbohydrate diet and a regime heavy on lunges, dead lifts, and single-leg leg presses, you have a combination that will round up your rear end just in time for summer!

And as for those vibration belts, don't waste your time.

86. Diuretics or water tablets will help you get lean

These contain mostly potassium, dandelion, uva ursi and caffeine (provided you purchased the legal, over-the-counter kind) and are meant to "flush out" several pounds of subcutaneous water during a 48-hour period thereby creating a lean and ripped physique for a short period of time. Does it work?

For 98% of all users, the answer is no. Let's look at the science behind it. Your body contains 80% water, which is stored in the inner organs, muscles, and under your skin. When you take a diuretic, the water comes from all sources, thereby flattening out your muscles and worsening your appearance.

Most people are also mistaken when it comes to their body composition. What is perceived as water is often fat, which simply needs to be burned off in order to achieve better definition. In other words, don't kid yourself: you need to diet. Also any potential benefit from the water loss would be extremely short-lived since being dehydrated is not a good position to be in.

There are, however, a few occasions when flushing out water makes sense, like a photo shoot or a bodybuilding ccmpetition. But even then, the benefits are questionable. If you are convinced that you are holding water, do a quick 20-minute whole body pump workout, this will pull the water from the under the skin into the muscle, helping you to appear more "cut". The bottom line is: If you are lean enough, you will look great regardless of any water you might be holding.

87. Green tea burns fat

This happens to be true, which explains why almost every fat burner these days contains green tea. First off, the active components of green tea such as EGCG, theanine and caffeine are very well researched with some 2,000-plus studies.
It is well known that caffeine has a good track record as a fat burner but that is not what makes green tea so special as a weight loss aid.

The interesting thing about green tea is that it works on different pathways. It may serve as a glucose regulator, since it slows the actions of amylase, which is an enzyme pivotal to the breakdown of carbohydrates. A controlled rise in blood sugar means there will be less of an insulin spike, which would reduce the fat storage after consuming carbs.

Green tea also inhibits fatty acid syntheses, which is an enzymatic system that stores carbohydrates as fat. A recent study, published in the *American Journal of Clinical Nutrition*, further validates green tea's effectiveness. The study indicated that drinking a tea rich in catechins (a major component of green tea extract) leads to both a lowering of body fat and of cholesterol levels. Furthermore, green tea reduces cardiovascular risks while helping you lose body fat. It is also one of the strongest antioxidants (like beta-carotene), some 200 times stronger than Vitamin E.

So this all sounds great and very scientific, but does it really burn fat at a noticeable rate?

It does, but don't expect earth-shattering results. Green tea is more of an overall health-promoting supplement with fat burning side benefits. If your diet and training are in check, green tea will give you an extra edge. You can find it in capsule form (make sure it says EGCG on the bottle) or make your own from fresh tea leaves. I prefer capsules since you would have to drink the equivalent of 10 cups per day to reap the full benefits.

88. Sports drinks are necessary during a workout

A lot of money is being made from drinks that "refuel" you or add a "plus" to your vitamin intake. But what use are they for the average trainee?

Not a whole lot, I am afraid. Electrolyte drinks make sense for athletes who train outside for several hours, such as cyclists, runners, and football players. Most people spend less than 1 hour in an air-conditioned gym; so there is no need for those extra calories, artificial sweeteners, and coloring agents. The vitamin/mineral balance of most of these drinks is also poorly laid out, usually consisting of some potassium, calcium, and vitamins C and B. Some of them also contain large amounts of high fructose corn syrup, which is definitely something you want to stay away from. If you are attempting to lose weight, any carbohydrate drink during the workout will stop fat oxidation in its tracks.

You will be fine just to supplement with water during your workout, especially if you are trying to lose weight. As for the vitamin supplementation, a simple multivitamin will provide you with a much broader range than any of these drinks.

Much greater importance should be placed on pre- and post-workout meals than on colorful sports drinks. These 2 or 3 meals might be the most crucial ones of the day since they provide the fuel for the workout and start your recovery quickly. When you work out, the nutrients in your bloodstream are those from the meal 1 to 2 hours before; any sports drink will still take 20 to 30 minutes to get into your system. In the rare case that you are about to perform a 2-hour workout, 10 grams of BCAAs or whey protein during the workout can help to fight catabolism.

This also makes your pre-workout meal your first line of recovery, followed by the post-workout intake. Here is a possible breakdown:

One hour before training:
Consume 50 grams of slow-digesting carbohydrates and 30 grams of protein. This could be a whole wheat bagel with some whey, a medium baked potato with 6 ounces of chicken, or tuna and whole wheat bread.

During workout:
12 to 20 ounces of water with BCAAs

Immediately after the workout:
Consume up to 0.5 grams of carbohydrates per each pound of bodyweight and 0.3 grams of protein per pound of body weight. For a 200-pound athlete that amounts to 100 grams of carbohydrates and 60 grams of protein. This meal is best taken in liquid form; grape juice and whey protein work very well. Studies have shown that this meal is critical for your recovery since it suppresses cortisol and kick starts the rebuilding process. One study has shown that this meal alone can shorten the recovery process by 24 hours.

One to 1.5 hours after the workout:
Another carbohydrate-protein meal—chicken and rice or tilapia and baked potatoes with some greens would work well.

As you can see, there is quite a heavy carbohydrate load around the workout. The reason is that the carbohydrates provide energy during the workout and the post workout insulin spike helps to shuttle nutrients into the muscle. The faster you replenish your depleted glycogen stores, the quicker you shift your body into muscle building gear.

If you are on a low carbohydrate diet, you need to skip the carbohydrates and add glutamine to your post workout drink. BCAAs before and during the workout can also help to stem catabolism.

89. Protein bars are good for you

They are so convenient, right? Thirty grams of protein; just unwrap and eat! Sounds too good to be true? It is.

Protein bars are certainly better than candy bars, since they contain a higher amount of protein and more vitamins, but this also where it ends.

Most bars have a high carbohydrates-to-protein ratio and are loaded with sugars, in some cases even HFCS. Label claims are also often inaccurate regarding the protein content. Some manufacturers add maltitol for sweetness and don't claim it as a carbohydrate, saying it has no influence on blood sugar levels.

Maltitol is a sugar alcohol and therefore a carbohydrate; its glycemic index is 52 (table sugar is 60), so it raises your blood sugar significantly. As for calories it delivers only 3 calories per gram as opposed to sugar, which has 4, but it does add calories to your daily intake.

Also, bars contain sweeteners, flavoring agents, and preservatives for a longer shelf life; not exactly the definition of clean foods.

So, when you are in a pinch, a protein bar is still an okay alternative, but try to not overuse them. Look for a bar that delivers as much protein as carbohydrates or at least a 1 to 1.5 ratio and scan the ingredients. If you find too many words like, maltodextrin, maltitol, or proprietary mixtures, stay away. As for the protein content, if the first words read calcium caseinate or soy protein, I would not recommend buying since those are inferior proteins.

Try to find a bar that is made primarily from oats, nuts, and whey protein and use it as a last resort meal when traveling.

90. Energy drinks before a workout give you an edge

Most energy drinks are a sugar and caffeine mix with a sprinkling of vitamins or ginseng. They tend to be very strongly flavored and colored. While it is true that the sugar/caffeine mix will create a short-term rush, there is also a crash at the end. What's more, you will be taking in a lot of empty calories plus unwanted chemicals. Excess caffeine consumption can also lead to a higher cortisol level in the blood, which will hinder your gains.

For your energy level, what you eat leading up to your workout is much more important. Try to consume 30 to 50 grams of complex carbohydrates with some 20 grams of protein 1 hour before the workout, drink sufficient water during the session, and crank up that iPod. If you really feel you need a boost, go with regular coffee or a caffeine pill; it's cheaper and won't be packed with sugars and chemicals.

Part V
Lifestyle

91. Stress and cortisol cause weight gain
92. The importance of sleep is overrated
93. I have never been in shape; so why should I believe I can do it now?
94. My job does not allow me to make gains
95. Bodybuilding requires me to be socially awkward, which means I can't do it
96. I am too old to get in shape
97. Vegetarians cannot build muscle
98. Organic food is better for you
99. I can drink alcohol and still build muscle and burn fat
10C.   I have a slow metabolism; that's why I am overweight
101.   I travel a lot, which makes it impossible to eat healthy

91.   Stress and cortisol cause weight gain

If you have watched infomercials, you have most likely seen the ads for cortisol-suppressing supplements. The sales pitch is simple: When you are stressed out, the body releases cortisol; cortisol stores water and fat (especially in the abdominal region); therefore you need a cortisol suppressor to make your belly disappear.

It seems to make sense, but it doesn't work. Cortisol is just the new bad boy of the fitness industry.

Every hormone in the human body has a purpose; no one hormone is inherently all good or all bad. Cortisol is a glandular hormone, excreted when a person is experiencing a fight or flight situation. It is the primary glucocorticoid, which means it increases the glucose levels in the blood stream. It also fights inflammation, in case you get injured or sick. You would have a hard time living without it.

Cortisol levels can be elevated due to strenuous dieting, training, travel, stress, and anger. This is not a bad thing, per se, since the hormone is needed to ensure proper bodily functions just like any other hormone in the system.

Cortisol does increase the storage of adipose tissue in the abdomen but only if provided with excess calories. The hormone itself cannot create energy out of thin air; it has to come from food.

Cortisol does, however, increase appetite. What's more, it creates a craving for calorie dense foods. Unfortunately, that particular mechanism is stronger than your conscience, which calls for healthy food and exercise. This combination then causes people with a high stress level to overeat or eat unconsciously. The result is weight gain. Alcohol consumption also tends to spike when there is a higher level of stress. If you don't get enough sleep because of work or family, it will take your body more metabolic work to function, which can then also cause additional hunger cravings.

Are there cortisol-suppressing supplements worth considering? There is little proof that any of them have much value for fat loss. It seems that Vitamin C, phosphatylserine, and glutamine might be your best bets if you feel you need to lower your cortisol levels. A good dosage would be 800 milligrams of phosphatylserine and 4,000 milligrams of Vitamin C.

What is much more important than any supplement, however, are stress levels. If they are high, there is a good chance that that will hinder your progress. Try to destress your life. Take a week off from training, get enough sleep, and maintain a healthy diet. Also, try to eliminate all stimulants, such as caffeine, for a while since they raise cortisol levels.

Stress is a huge energy drain. You can't have stress if you want to lose that belly fat and build muscle.

No pill will do that for you.

92.   The importance of sleep is overrated

If anything, sleep is underrated. Eight hours of sleep is a must and an afternoon nap is even better. If you deprive yourself of sleep, not only does your recovery suffer but you also create a hormonal imbalance, which will greatly hinder your gains in the gym.

During the deep sleep phase, the majority of your body's growth hormone (GH) is being released. One week of sleep-disturbed nights can cause your body to secrete less growth hormone and more cortisol than you need. High cortisol levels in the body can lead to fat gain and the lower growth hormone will make it harder to lose adipose tissue. People who don't get enough sleep tend to eat unconsciously all through the day. Your concentration will suffer, which will affect workout performance negatively and heighten your risk of injury.

Rest allows protein synthesis (the repair and rebuilding of muscle damage inflicted by training), which gives your muscles a chance to grow. Without rest you can't repair the damage done in the gym. You can enhance the muscle repair process by consuming a whey shake with peanut butter or flax seed oil before retiring.

To make maximum progress you need as much sleep as possible. Beware though, if you are one of those rare individuals with unlimited time, there is such a thing as too much sleep. Try to keep it to 12 hours a day, but I don't think this is a huge concern for most people

If you struggle with getting enough sleep, there are a few good herbal remedies: St. John's Wort, passionflower, valerian root, and melatonin. A cocktail made from 3 milligrams of melatonin, 500 milligrams of passion flower and 1 gram of valerian root should work for most people.

93. I have never been in shape; so why should I believe I can do it now?

Because the choice is up to you.

The majority of cells in the body are being replaced every 6 months, so the things you ate at the last company outing are long gone. Your body is bound to react to training and nutrition; it is biology 101. If a muscle is confronted with a new form of stress, it will respond by growing stronger. If your fat deposits are needed as energy to heal the muscle tears incurred through training, they will shrink.

The key to success is a proper plan with bi-weekly goals. Reaching those goals will keep you motivated as you progress. If you feel that you need assistance, hire a qualified person who can help you outline such a plan. Make sure you don't have injuries or other conditions that might interfere with your training program.

Next, go food shopping. The truly nutritious items in the supermarket, such as greens, dairy, eggs, lean meats, and all-natural nut butters, are in the side aisles. So shop on the sides only.

Lastly, don't overdo it. Beginners who are too impatient run the risk of burning out. Try to get to the gym 2 to 3 times a week and work hard to improve every time, as opposed to just amassing "garbage time" (time spent in the gym where you don't make any progress with regard to weight lifted and sets or reps performed).

Nothing is standing in between you and your new body but your excuses. Don't let them stop you.

94. My job does not allow me to stick to diet and exercise

It all comes down to making training and proper eating a priority. Even if you can get in only 1 workout during the week, that still leaves 2 for the weekend. In a worst-case scenario, 2 whole body workouts or a push/pull routine will still produce sufficient progress. Some people even make better gains on drastically reduced volume.

Stick with basic exercises such as squats, dead lifts, incline bench press, bent over rows, pull ups and try to improve either your weights or rep numbers on every workout.

It is important to keep a training log so you can strive for a 2 to 5% increase in weights every week. Challenge yourself during the workouts. You can add partial repetitions at the end of the set or change your grip or stance in order to create a new stimulus.

With regard to diet, most work places have a refrigerator where you can store cottage cheese, grilled chicken, etc. Rice cakes, oats, and almonds don't even need cooling, and most lunch options can be customized for your needs. Vegetables can be bought already chopped up so they are easier to eat.

You should also have 2 cooking days per week. Make 12 to 14 portions of the meals you need and store them in Tupperware in your fridge or in the office.

If your job requires you to travel a lot, a cooler should become your new best friend, since you can store several meals in t. Steel mugs can be helpful for your protein shakes. Other staples are nuts, apples, beef jerky, and protein bars.

95. Bodybuilding requires me to be socially awkward, which means I can't do it

This is an excuse you often hear from people who never really tried to make a healthy lifestyle work for them. Now, in all fairness, getting and staying in shape requires a certain amount of dedication and discipline and can at times cause complications in a social setting.

Proper planning goes a long way in that regard. Don't let your meals become haphazard. If you are not sure where you are going to be, cook ahead and take your meals with you.

Schedule times for your workouts and stick to them. If you have to go back to the office afterwards, fine. You might even be more productive since you cleared your head and are ful of endorphins. If this doesn't work for you, then you can work out before going to work. This can be a drag during winter, but if you get it done early you don't have to worry about it during the day. Studies show that people who get their workout in before going to work are more likely to stick with their routine.

Staying dedicated to your diet and exercise plan will sometimes force you to make choices that others won't understand (why won't you have another drink? Why can't you eat lasagna?) But the truth is that in our society "normal" sometimes does not mean healthy, so stick to your guns.

Of course, we all must find a way to exist within society, so don't make yourself a hermit either. The world won't come to an end if you eat a slice of pie on Thanksgiving, just don't eat it every day between Thanksgiving and New Years!

96.   I am too old to get in shape

In a society where youth seems to be the highest good and anyone over 25 is essentially on his or her way to pureed foods and bingo afternoons, some people feel that they've missed their window to get in shape.

I can tell you from my experience as a trainer that this is simply not true. Let's take a look at what happens as we age: testosterone and growth hormone decline, which makes it harder to recover and build muscle. Metabolism slows down, so fat loss takes longer. And lastly, the joints and ligaments become less stable; so you are more prone to injury.

Wow, that's depressing. So maybe you should just throw in the towel, watch movies, and eat nachos with cheese dip since all is lost? No need; in fact, all the above-mentioned processes can be at least partially reversed through proper training and nutrition. Resistance training increases your hormonal levels and elevates your metabolism significantly, as does a high protein diet with a good amount of essential fats and complex carbohydrates. Joints and ligaments also get stronger if challenged by a weight workout. There are, however, a few things you should consider if you're over 40:

1. Train less than you used to. Chances are you are over-trained as it is, so you must reduce the number of sets or sessions but not the intensity so your body can recover from the workouts.
2. Set goals every 4 to 6 weeks. There is no one routine for all, always push yourself hard and take stock after 6 weeks. If it doesn't work, change it.
3. Pay very close attention to nutrition. You need 5 to 6 clean meals in order to achieve your physique goals.

4. Take a supplement like glucosamine/chondroitin for joint health.
5. Rest! Try to sleep 7 to 8 hours a night. If you can nap, even better.
6. Get help with recovery. Massages, yoga classes, and sauna—all these things can make a difference in your performance.

Also, regardless of your starting age, you can always dramatically improve your physique. Don't be fooled by the myth that you need to be 18 to get in shape—start lifting!

97. Vegetarians cannot build muscle

It is often said that vegetarians don't consume sufficient amounts of protein, minerals, and healthy fats needed to build muscle.

However, if you look at the physiques of vegetarian body builders Bill Pearl or Andreas Cahling, you certainly don't see any muscular deficiencies. It's all about making sure you get the food and nutrients you need. For iron, zinc, calcium, and potassium, vegetarians should consume broccoli, wheat germ, oranges, bananas, spinach, and peanut butter. The only vitamin that could be problematic is B-12, since it is only found in animal products. Here a B-12 supplement would be useful (20-50 mcg for most adults). Vegetarians should also make sure they get Omega 3 fatty acids by eating soy, walnuts, avocados, coconut oil, and olive oil.

For bodybuilders, the single biggest issue is eating enough protein. The fact that vegetarians don't consume many of the common proteins—animal products—means it is hard to consume high quality protein.

While it is true that animal proteins are superior in biological value to their plant counterparts, there are also ways to ensure that a vegetarian consumes enough high-quality protein to ensure muscle growth. The challenge is that in order to achieve their protein requirements, vegetarians would have to eat large amounts of food since beans, nuts, and soy beans do not deliver a lot of protein per portion. But this can be solved with either supplements or making smart food choices.

How to stay anabolic as a vegetarian

For vegetarians soy protein is one the best weapons they have. Soy is high quality protein with similar properties to whey and a good amount of glutamine. Its fast digestibility makes it a great pre- or post-workout protein.

For those that are not vegan, eggs, low-fat cheese, and whey protein are great choices and will make for a very powerful muscle-building stack.

For vegans, there is also hope. Since we live in the 21st century, science has come up with some great plant-based proteins such as soy, rice, hemp, pea, and buckwheat. Buckwheat protein has been all the rage recently due to its high bioavailability and biological value. It has the most complete amino acid chain of any grain-based protein and seems to have cholesterol-lowering abilities.

Supplementation with the aforementioned products will satisfy a vegetarian's protein needs without adding the extra carbohydrates that come from protein-rich foods like peas, soy beans, and rice. This will come in very handy when dieting.

One of the nutritional mantras for vegetarians used to be: rice and beans together make a complete protein so always combine the two in a dish. This is not true, however, since you have a steady pool of amino acids (about 20-30 grams) in your body. As long as you consume both foods during the day you will be fine. Your body will simply use the amino acids in the blood stream to find the missing amino acids.

If you're still worried about your protein intake, just add a scoop of whey with all meals to ensure optimal biological availability.

Even non-vegetarians should consider implementing a non-animal based protein into their diet in order to prevent the body from getting used to your everyday proteins.

Variety is key!

98.   Organic food is better for you

Organic food is all the rage these days and the price difference between organic and nonorganic foods is shrinking. So does it make sense to eat organic?

For the most part it holds true, but a distinction needs to be made. The nutritional value of organic food is often not a lot higher than that of its conventional competitors. But the amount of additives you don't want to eat, such as pesticides, steroids, growth hormones, and antibiotics, is much less.

If you can afford it, try to consume organic milk and meat. These two foods in particular in their nonorganic forms can be laced with hormones; so spending the extra money on organic is worth it. Organic eggs from free range and grain fed chickens are also worth the trouble since they contain more Omega 3 fatty acids than regular ones (especially interesting when you are low carbing).

As for vegetables and fruit, you can buy the nonorganic versions of anything with a thick skin, such as avocados or oranges, since you don't plan to eat the outside. Organically and locally grown corn and tomatoes, on the other hand, can contain up to 50% less pesticides and 30% more nutrients.

Another thing to consider might be to buy locally. The shorter the transport the more nutrients you're likely to find in your produce. Plus, you are helping the local farmers. Many cities have 100-mile clubs to help you locate stores and markets that sell local produce.

99. I can drink alcohol and still build muscle and burn fat

Not a lot, I am afraid. Alcohol is one of the biggest monkey wrenches you can throw at your system. It derails your muscle building and fat burning train on several counts. First, alcohol delivers a lot of empty calories; in fact alcohol contains 7 calories per gram as opposed to protein or carbohydrates, which have 4. Alcohol is also the first fuel that the body burns, which stops any fat loss. Imagine a highway with the President passing through. As long as Mr. Obama's motorcade is on the highway, no other car will drive there. The same holds true for alcohol in your body: unless it is burned off as acetate, the body will not tap into the fat reserves for energy. This takes up to 12 hours; so if someone consumes several drinks on different nights a week, that person will only have 4 out of 7 days for fat loss. You can see where I am going with this.

Alcohol tends to get stored as visceral fat, which is a layer of fat wrapped around your organs thereby causing the so-called beer belly.

Since alcohol loosens inhibition and stimulates the appetite, many people overeat when they drink, creating an even higher caloric uptake. To make matters worse, most drinking establishments don't exactly provide a clean eating menu (pizza and chicken fingers, anyone?)

Alcohol also suppresses testosterone, thereby lowering the metabolic rate and eliminating testosterone as a muscle builder. Less testosterone means less muscle, which can cause a higher amount of fat to be stored.

Lastly, alcohol inhibits your athletic performance. You simply won't be able train hard after consuming several alcoholic beverages. The symptoms are decreased strength, impaired coordination and increased fatigue. Since the effect lasts 48 hours, consuming alcohol twice a week, leads to a loss of 4 days of training during that week.

If you must drink alcohol, pick one day a week and stick with red wine, beer or on the rocks drinks. Being German, I would recommend the wheat beers such as Weihenstephan or Franziskaner, since they don't contain any preservatives or coloring agents. Stay away from high sugar content mixed drinks and limit your consumption to 2 drinks. Always have a glass of water with you and keep your drink in the non-dominant hand. This will help you to drink less.

If you want to get the most out of your training, I would recommend staying away from alcohol altogether. The same goes for anyone on a low carbohydrate diet, since alcohol makes it harder to stay in ketosis.

Save the glass of wine for your carbohydrate meal to stay sane!

100. I have a slow metabolism; that's why I am overweight

"I know this person who eats pizza and donuts all the time without gaining weight. I wish I had his metabolism."

When all diet and training efforts fail, the problem must be metabolism, right? Not quite. Sadly, your parents were wrong; you are NOT different. Everyone on this earth has to follow the same laws of physics, which determine the balance of the energy.

In all fairness, there is a small percentage of people who suffer from hypothyroidism or low thyroid function, which can cause weight gain. If you think you might fall into this group, have your doctor test your hormone levels.

Then there is another small percentage of the population that is so-called "diet-resistant," meaning their metabolism adapts quicker to the change in caloric intake and fights back harder to avoid weight loss. They can still gain or lose weight but at a slower pace.

No one can beat the universe

Ok, enough excuses, on to the other 6 billion people. No one can beat the universe, which in this case is the law of thermodynamics as it pertains to your personal energy balance.

Any energy you store, be it muscle or fat (unfortunately, it's often the latter) had to be consumed at some point. It is impossible to make something out of nothing. If you could do that, you would be able to fix the world's hunger problem and relieve us of our oil dependence while you're at it. If you eat 100 calories, that is the maximum you can store—they can't magically turn into 800 calories.

So one reason for the slow metabolism myth is that people are extremely bad at counting calories. They grossly underestimate what they eat and overestimate the amount of energy burned, which leads them to conclude that it must be their metabolism that is slow and not the energy balance.

However, we are not all completely equal; there are small differences in metabolisms.

What constitutes metabolism?

Let's look at what metabolism really is in order to better understand the dilemma. Every living being needs a constant supply of energy in order to perform physical and mental activities. This energy is converted out of matter (food); the more energy a person needs on a daily basis, the higher this person's basic metabolic rate (BMR) will be.

Now while it is true that some people have a higher BMR than others, the difference is not big enough to make a person overweight. From top (super fast) to bottom (super slow) there is only a 10 to 15% difference. This sounds like a lot but let's break it down into numbers. Let's assume we have two dieters and we establish their caloric needs at 1,500 calories per day. Both are now put on a 1,000 calorie-per-day diet. It then turns out that dieter B is on the super slow side so his BMR is really only 1,350 calories. However, at a 1,000 calorie per day he should still lose weight, albeit at a slower pace than his 1,500-calorie per day counterpart.

The same holds true for the metabolic slowdown during the diet. Your metabolism might slow down 10%, but if the deficit is 30%, you will still lose weight.

What about your friend who eats pizza and ice cream without ever gaining weight? Chances are he doesn't eat junk all the time, and his brain is more efficient in blunting his appetite.

What really constitutes someone's BMR is body composition or the relationship between fat and muscle mass. Someone with more muscle mass has a faster metabolism than someone who stores a lot of body fat since fat burns very few calories. So, as you can see, overweight people have a slower BMR because they tend to be less physically active and carry more body fat, not the other way around.

A NEAT way to speed things up

That brings us to one of the few variables in BMR among people: NEAT, or Non-Exercises Activity Thermogenesis. This covers everything from making phone calls to standing to walking to working. In essence, fidgeting. The amount of calories burned can range anywhere from 200 to 700 a day, which adds up. Lean people often seem like the Energizer bunny, constantly on the move, jumping, gesticulating, etc. If you struggle with your weight, try to emulate some of those ideas. Take the stairs, stand up at the computer, take walks every 30 minutes; all these small activities will add up to significant weight loss.

Most caffeine containing fat burners help with that, because they give people a boost of energy, which makes them move more.

Other ways to speed up your metabolism

The other two contributors to your energy balance are the thermic effect of exercise (TEE) and the thermic effect of food (TEF).

Let's cover TEF first and how this can be useful to you?

First and foremost, eat breakfast! A wholesome meal in the morning will prevent your body from shutting down and going into starvation mode. Eating several high protein meals is another must to keep your metabolism high since protein works as a thermogenic. Cinnamon, ginger, and cayenne pepper also have an effect on your body's temperature.

Drinking lots of water is helpful because the conversion of matter into energy can't happen without water. About 75% of America is constantly dehydrated. Dehydration is often mistaken for hunger, which then leads to excess calorie intake. Whenever you think that you are hungry, drink 10 ounces of water. If within 10 minutes you are still hungry, eat something.

And for the TEE, there is working out. Cardio works well as an energy expenditure and of course, there is weight training—which is the best form of exercise for raising your BMR. Resistance training builds muscle, which will then elevate your BMR at all times, not just while working out.

So the idea of a slow metabolism is merely an excuse (a small part of the population aside); don't let it stand between you and your beach body!

101. I travel a lot, which makes it impossible to eat healthy

Here I feel like something of an expert, as it is not uncommon for me to chase all over Manhattan during the day, eating most of my meals on the subway (a sad state of affairs, I know).

Traveling can indeed be stressful on your diet, but it doesn't have to be disastrous. Different time zones, limited choices, and meetings make it difficult to always find grilled chicken and brown rice.

Does that mean you are excused, and we'll meet at the Dunkin' Donuts counter? Not at all. It just means that you will have to plan a little more. When traveling by plane, bring your own food. Airport terminals have gotten a lot better in terms of what is available. It's not difficult to find nuts, protein bars, and salads with grilled chicken. If you don't want to rely on other people, bring almonds, rice cakes, and protein powder with you as well as plenty of water. The humidity in airplanes can drop to 10%, which is an arid environment. Make sure you stay hydrated; it will also help with the jetlag.

For the road warrior, there are more possibilities to store food in your car. You might even consider purchasing a small cooler to bring whole meals. If you are stranded at one of the many fast food places along the highway, don't despair. Their menus have improved a lot over recent years; even KFC now has grilled chicken. While there still tends to be a lot of sodium, the ban of trans fats has worked wonders for the overall nutritional content of these places.

Almost all of them carry some sort of grilled meat and vegetables. As for salads, beware: some of them come with dressing and croutons, which can add hundreds of extra calories. (Taco Bell's fully loaded salads come to 970 calories!) Be very careful or simply get a burger and toss the bun. Try to order a baked potato or steamed vegetables instead of fries or mashed potatoes on the side.

Sandwiches are to be avoided. While some may claim to be low in fat, they contain up to 70 grams of carbohydrates and very little protein in the processed meats inside (and that is without the chips and soda).

I have compiled a list of the most common fast food places you will find at most US airports and picked 1 or 2 meals with around 35 to 50 grams of protein, 40 grams of carbohydrates, and 10 to 15 grams of fat you can choose from:

Starbucks: Order the power protein breakfast called the protein plate. If you have just worked out, you can use one of their yogurt parfaits to replenish your muscle glycogen.
McDonald's: Premium Caesar Salad with grilled chicken, dressing on the side, or the grilled chicken sandwich with half a bun.
KFC: Roasted Chicken Caesar Salad without dressing, Tender Roast Sandwich without Sauce (perfect for after a workout).
Burger King: Tendergrill Chicken Sandwich if you need the carbohydrates, or Tendergrill Chicken Salad if low-carbing

IHop: Spinach, mushroom, and tomato omelet or simply grilled chicken sandwich. The balsamic glazed chicken sandwich also works, though the protein content is a bit lower.

Wendy's: Mandarin Chicken Salad; add almonds if you want more fats. Adding a plain baked potato would make it a great post-workout choice. Another option would be the Ultimate Grilled Chicken Sandwich. Wendy's also offers you the choice to order a la carte, e.g., getting just a hamburger patty with a baked potato.

Jamba Juice: Caesar salad, no dressing is a good choice if you are low carbing. Gobble'licious sandwich could be used after a workout. I would stay away from all their smoothies since they contain a lot of carbohydrates. One exception is the Protein Berry Whey, which could be used before a workout.

Subway: Roast beef mini sub or all salads without dressing. The sodium content is somewhat high but that won't matter hugely unless you have a photo shoot or a bodybuilding contest the next day (in which case you should be carrying your own foods in the first place).

Boston market: They serve a wide variety of whole meals such as a one-quarter white meat chicken; baked beans or fresh steamed vegetables would work as a side.

Pizza hut: Two slices of the Fit'n Delicious Pizza with all-natural chicken

Popeye's: Grilled chicken breast, skin removed with a bowl of red beans and rice or Cajun rice if you can handle the carbohydrates; otherwise stick with green beans as a side.

White Castle: Two to three Golden Chicken Breast sandwiches, no bun.

Arby's: Regular roast beef or chopped Farmhouse grilled chicken salad.

Dunkin' Donuts: Turkey cheese sandwich or a whole grain bagel with some whey protein.

Taco Bell: Fresco Burritos Supreme, chicken as well as steak.

Quiznos: Their small sandwiches are decent, Chicken Carbonara or Black Angus steak, for example. Just get them without cheese or dressing.

Blimpie: If you need the carbohydrates, go with a 6-inch Chicken Teriyaki; if you don't, the buffalo chicken salad is a good alternative.

Gas stations almost always carry some protein bars, nuts, and beef jerky as well as milk for a quick high-protein snack. At vending machines, you should be able to get nuts or whole-wheat crackers.

It is crucial that you never let yourself go really hungry. Hunger leads to muscle loss and overeating. So always carry some small snacks such as nuts with you in order to avoid hunger pangs (this might be the chance for protein bars to shine).

Traveling certainly makes it harder to eat healthy but it shouldn't be an excuse. With a little bit of planning you can stay on track.

Appendix: Physique Building To-Go

Weight lifting training systems

5x5: a training system to primarily develop strength and mass, popularized by Bill Starr. It is often used in the football off-season and is centered around the big three exercises: squat, dead lift and bench press. The goal is to improve performance 3 to 5% a week over a 6-week cycle. Each exercise is trained with 5 sets of reps and variable loads.

8x8: The brainchild of Vince Gironda, the athlete performs 8 sets of 8 reps with very short breaks (20 seconds). A great tool to shock the body and improve definition.

100s: here the athlete performs 100 reps per exercise. Pick a weight that is about 50% your regular training weight, you should be able to perform 40-plus reps at a time, rest 1 second for each rep you fall short, then continue until you hit 100. Do as many sets as needed. It's a great system for a shock week.

HST: hypertrophy specific training by Bryan Haycock, the athlete performs up to 3 full-body workouts a week with increasing loads and decreasing rep numbers over a 6-week cycle.

HIT: high intensity training by Mike Mentzer and Arthur Jones, the trainee does only 1 set per exercise to absolute failure and trains only every fifth day. The focus is on recovery and intensity.

Split routine: The body is split in several body parts and each part is trained once a week. Example: chest and arms, back and shoulders, legs. One of the most popular ways to train.

POF: position of flexion, developed by Steve Holeman, each muscle is trained in midrange, stretch, and contracted position. Example: triceps: dips, mid range, overhead extensions for the stretch, and press downs for the contracted position.

GVT: German volume training, here the athlete performs 10 sets of 10 reps with a rather high load. Often done in an alternating style.

> Example:
> A: 10x10 of bench press
> B: 10x10 pull ups
> Perform 1 set of A, rest 2 minutes, do 1 set of B, etc

Cardio routines

Low intensity: long cardio sessions with a heart rate of about 130 bpm, 30-40 minutes.
HIIT: high intensity interval training, where the athlete warms up at a moderate pace for 5 minutes and then performs 5 to 7 sprints of 30-45 seconds with 1 minute rest in between, The goal is to increase EPOC (excess postexercise oxygen consumption).

The most popular cutting diets

Low carb diet: the majority of calories come from fat and protein, carbs are only eaten 1 to 2 times a week.
Low fat diet: carbs are eaten every day, but the fat content of the diet is usually kept around 10%.
Ketogenic diet: very low carb diet, with the goal of putting the athlete into ketosis, where the body burns fat for fuel.
Zig Zag diet: calories and carb intake are varied from day to day while still achieving a weekly caloric deficit
      Example:
      Monday high carb,
      Tuesday low carb,
      Wednesday no carbs,
      Thursday no carbs,
      Friday high carb,
      Saturday and Sunday low-carb days

Appendix: Five Exercises Everyone Must Do

Building a great physique should not be complicated (please note, I did not say it is easy). Most trainees overcomplicate things by following high-volume routines, which only lead to frustration. This is not necessary! If you master these 5 exercises and work on them diligently, in conjunction with a well planned diet, you will make amazing progress.

Squat

Some people call it the king of all exercises, and there is some truth to it. Squats are a full body workout in themselves—it takes more than 200 muscles to squat. Done properly, they will build your legs as well as abs and lower back. They will also improve your cardiovascular health and improve your respiratory capacity.
Execution: 1. Step under the bar with a shoulder width stance, feet pointed outward. Raise the bar on your shoulders, take one step back, inhale, contract the abs and look up.
Collapse from the hips first as you initiate the downward movement, then the knees will follow. Make sure not to lean forward at the bottom of the squat, push your chest out, and squat back up.
Squat as deep as you are comfortable; always push from the heels of your feet, never the toes.

Deadlift

This is a fantastic full-body exercise, which will develop core strength (great for relieving back pain). In addition to lower back and mid back, the deadlift builds strength in the hamstrings, quads, glutes, traps, calves, and forearms
Execution: With the bar racked ideally at mid shin, stand close to the bar and grip it at shoulder width. Lower your glutes, look up, and exhale. Begin to pull the bar up along your legs until you stand erect. Lower in the same fashion. NEVER let the bar dangle in front of you or look down.

Standing barbell press

The standing barbell press will take care of your shoulders and triceps development. What's more, since you are standing, you will have to engage your abdominal muscles during the entire exercise.

Execution: Assume a shoulder wide stance under the bar and grip the bar about 2 inches wider than your shoulders. Tighten the abs, lift the bar off of the rack, exhale, and push up. Lower the bar to the chin, repeat. NEVER press form behind the head.

Incline bench press or dips

As mentioned before, I do not like the flat bench as a pec builder. Incline bench or dips will work great to develop front delts, chest and triceps.

Execution for the incline press: Lie down on an incline bench (angle no more than 40 degrees); make sure your feet, hips, and shoulder blades are on the floor/bench. Grip the bar a little bit outside your shoulders, pinch your shoulder blades together, and lower the bar slowly until it is about a fist above the chest. Exhale and push up.

Execution for dips: assume a wide grip; place your feet behind you so you can lean forward. Keep your chin tucked to the chest as you lower yourself. Exhale and push up.

Bent over rows or pull ups

To finish up, you get to work your lats and biceps. This is done with a pulling exercise; vary your grip (wider or narrower), depending on which part of your back you want to train. I recommend changing it up weekly. Both exercises also provides stimulus for the forearms and abs.

Execution for the bent over row: Here it is best to imagine yourself as a crane. Stand over the bar, grip it at shoulder width, and pull to your lower abs while looking ahead. Don't look down ever. The upper body does not move; only the arms are pulling up the weight.

Execution for the pull up: Choose any grip you like (parallel is most suitable for beginners); start by contracting the shoulder blades and pull yourself up to the bar. Inhale while lowering.

GLOSSARY

1st law of thermodynamics: energy can be transferred but never created or destroyed

1 RM: 1 rep max, the maximum weight someone can lift with 1 repetition

ACL: anterior crucial ligament

Adipose tissue: stored fat

Adrenoreceptors: cells in the body, who couple with adrenaline and nor adrenaline. They can inhibit or block lypolysis

Amino acids: building blocks of protein

Amylase: enzyme responsible for the break down of carbohydrates

Anabolic: muscle building

ATP: adenosine tri phosphate, energy stored in cell, derived from creatine

BCAAs: branched chain amino acids, namely valine, leucine and isoleucine. Helpful in stopping muscle wasting during training

Biological availability of protein or biological value (BV): measures how much muscle the body can build out of 100 grams ingested protein. The reference point is the egg with 100.

Bodybuilding: changing your body, can be gaining muscle, lose fat or both

Training: improving your capacity to work, in regards to weight training to strive to either move more weight, take shorter rests or perform more reps with the same weight

BMR: basic metabolic rate, the amount of energy you use during 24 hours of absolute rest

Bulking: overeating with the goal to put on muscle

CNS: central nervous system

Cortisol: anti-inflammatory, muscle wasting (catabolic) hormone

Compound exercise: any exercise, which requires several muscles and joints to work in an integrated manner. Squats, rows, dead lifts, presses

Cutting: undereating to lose fat and 'lean out"

CYP34A: liver enzyme, which is responsible for the break down of caffeine

Diet: your nutritional intake, contrary to popular belief it does not have a time limit. If you want to have a great physique you need to eat accordingly all the time

DHA: Docosahexaenoic Acid, also found in fish oil

DNP: 2-4 dinitrophenol, fat burner derived from TNT, highly dangerous

Droopy chest: a chest that appears saggy

Ectomorph: 1 of the 3 soma types typically has long limbs, narrow shoulders and hips as well as a fast metabolism. Doesn't gain muscle easily but stays lean

EFA: essential fatty acids

EPA: Eicosapentaenoic acid, essential fatty acids found in fish oil

EGCG: Epigallocatechin gallat, active ingredient in green tea

EPOC: exercise post oxygen consumption or after burn effect

Ergogenic: any external aids that can improve performance

Ez bar: easy bar or cambered bar

Fascia: connective tissue, which surrounds the muscles of the body

FFA: free form fatty acids, fatty acids that have been oxidized and can be used for energy

Flavonoid: compounds found in fruit

GH: growth hormone

Gluconeogenesis: the creation of glucose from non-glucose sources, fatty acids etc

Glycemic index: tool to measure the insulin response of foods, reference point is table sugar with 100.

Glycogen stores: carbohydrates, stored in muscle and liver, used as energy during training.

HFCS: high fructose corn syrup, industrial sweetener

hGH: human Growth Hormone

Hypertrophy: muscle growth

IGF-1: insulin like Growth factor, powerful muscle building hormone

Insulin: storage hormone, responsible for the transport of nutrients, storage of glucose in the muscle.

Insulin resistance: cells have become resistant against insulin, this reduces the effectiveness on insulin, increases fat storage while reducing the effectiveness in storing glycogen

Isolation exercise: requires only one joint, such as biceps curl

IT band: iliotibial band, stretches from hip to the knee on the outside of the leg

Junking out: have a binge meal consisting of junk food

Lipase: Enzyme, which helps with lypolysis

Lipolysis: fat oxidation or break down of fats stored in a fat cell

Maltitol: sugar alcohol

Maltodextrin: simple sugar

Mesomorph: somatype, broad shoulders, small waist, gains muscle easy

Mind-muscle connection: being able to effectively feel the muscle while training, not just moving the weights

Mono-and disaccharide: simple sugars

Myofascial release: soft tissue therapy, in order to release pressure and pain on certain muscles and ligaments. Can be done on foam roll

NEAT: non-exercise thermogenic activity

Neural output: the ability to contract your muscles effectively during training

Neuromuscular efficiency: *see neural output*

Neural fatigue: one of the symptoms of overtraining, often accompanied by loss of appetite and moodiness

Norepinephedrine: a stress hormone, secreted by the adrenal glands, that helps with fat loss

NSAID (non-steroidal anti-inflammatory drug): aspirin, Motrin, Tylenol

Nutrition partitioning: the process by which ingested calories get stored as either muscle or fat

Overtraining: pushing your body too hard thereby reaching a state where muscle is lost and fat is gained despite training. Symptoms are: elevated pulse rate, loss of appetite, strength loss, irritability, and sleeplessness
If that occurs, take 10 days off and increase your calories.

Testosterone: male sex hormone, muscle building

Pecs: pectoral (chest) muscles

Phytonutrients: components in plants thought to promote health

Polysaccharide: complex carbohydrate

Pro athlete: performs a sport for a living

Protein synthesis: the process of repairing protein and building muscle on a cellular level

Quad sweep: placing more emphasis on the outer part of the quadriceps to create a more *sweeping* appearance

RICE (rest, ice, compress, elevate): recommended treatment for ankle injuries

Subcutaneous fat: fat found under the skin

SNS: sympathetic nervous system

Spot reduction: the myth that one can reduce body fat in one area by training a particular muscle

T-3 and T-4: thyroid hormones that regulate your metabolic rate, the amount of energy you need during the day

TEE (thermic effect of exercise): the amount of calories burned during a workout session

TEF (thermic effect of food): amount of energy it takes to digest a certain food

TFL (tensor fascia late): helps to abduct thigh and flex hips

Thermogenesis: heat production in the body

Visceral fat: internal layer of fat surrounding the organs, creates the beer belly

Visualization: technique for establishing a connection with a muscle in order to train it more effectively. Usually done via contracting and relaxing

VO2 max: maximum oxygen uptake or the maximum capacity of someone's body to transport oxygen

Water retention: film of water under the skin, causes loss of muscle definition. Can be caused by sodium, lactose, or stress

Select Bibliography and Further Reading

The books and articles here are all either standard works in their respective fields or provide a new perspective. I do not agree with all the findings, but I believe it is necessary to present both sides in order to form an educated opinion.

Berardi, John and Michael Meji. *Scrawny to Brawny: The Complete Guide to Building Muscle the Natural Way*. Emmaus, PA: Rodale Books, 2005.
A great book for the natural trainee, with detailed workouts and meal plans.

Bompa, Tudor and Lorenzo Cornacchia. *Serious Strength Training*. Champaign, Ill: Human Kinetics Publishers, 1998.
Pretty much the standard work on weight training, Tudor Bompa is one of the pioneers of periodization training.

Cordain, Loren and Joe Friel. *The Paleo Diet For Athletes: A Nutritional Formula for Peak Athletic Performance*. Emmaus, Penn: Rodale Books, 2005.
The book stirred a lot of controversy, since it goes against the grain (literally) but it delivers a well thought out approach toward diet.

McDonald, Lyle. *The Protein Book: A Complete Guide for the Athlete and Coach*. Taylorsville, UT: Lyle McDonald Publishing, 2007.
Good guide for anyone who is interested in the nuts and bolts of protein.

McDonald, Lyle. *The Ultimate Diet 2.0*. Taylorsville, UT: Lyle McDonald Publishing, 2003.
Not an easy diet but it works, also gives great background information.

McDonald, Lyle. *The Rapid Fat Loss Handbook, second edition*. Taylorsville, UT: Lyle McDonald Publishing, 2008.
Also not an easy diet but effective and very useful for the background information.

Gironda, Vince. *The Wild Physique: The Complete Book of Championship Training for Men and Women*. Mississauga, Canada: Musclemag International,1975.
The iron guru himself wrote it, a must-have. Vince Gironda trained every star from Clint Eastwood to Cher in the 70's.

Holeman, Steve and Jonathan Lawson. *Beyond X-Rep*. Oxnard, Calif: Ironman Magazine, 2005.
Interesting approach to mass building, especially for natural trainees.

Holeman, Steve and Jonathan Lawson. *The Ultimate Mass Workout*. Oxnard, Calif: Ironman Magazine, 2004.

Holeman, Steve and Jonathan Lawson. *X-traordinary Arms*. Oxnard, Calif: Ironman Magazine, 2007.
Great breakdown of the anatomy of the arm plus different workouts.

Llewllyn, William. *Anabolics 2005*. Jupiter, FL: Body of Science, 2005.
Llewllyn approaches this controversial topic in the most objective matter while staying away from under- or overestimating the dangers of these drugs.

Willey, Warren. *Better than Steroids*. Bloomington, IN: Trafford Publishing, 2007.
Interesting read with regard to postworkout nutrition and different diet approaches.

Schuler, Lou, Cassandra Forsythe, and Alwyn Cosgrove. *The New Rules of Lifting for Women: Lift Like a Man, Look Like a Goddess*. New York: Avery Trade, 2007.
One of the best lifting books written expressly for women.

Rudolph, Chuck. *Game Over: The Final Showtime Cut Diet You'll Ever Need!* (volume 2). Scivation Books, 2006.
Easy-to-follow keto diet.

Schwarzenegger, Arnold with Bill Dobbins. *Encyclopedia of Modern Bodybuilding*. Pelham Practical Sports, 1985.
Arnold made bodybuilding; if nothing else, buy it for the photos.

Duchaine, Dan. *Underground Bodyopus: Militant Weight Loss and Recomposition.* Xipe Press, 1996.
A pioneer work with regard to to refeeds and keto diets.

Darden, Ellington and Mike Mentzer. *The Nautilus Bodybuilding Book.* Chicago Ill: Contemporary Books, 1982.
Good history of HIT, with emphasis on the recovery aspect of training

Delavier, Frederic. *Strength Training Anatomy, second edition.* Champaign, Ill: Human Kinetics, 2005.
One of the most detailed anatomy books with regard to strength training.

Poliquin, Charles. *Modern Trends in Strength Training, Volume 1: Sets and Reps.* Charlespoliquin.net, 2001.
Poliquin, Charles. *Winning the Arms Race.* Charlespoliquin.net, 2001
Poliquin's athletes have won more than 25 Olympic medals.

Stoppani, Jim. "The Nutrition Notebook: How Do You Like Them Apples?" *Muscle and Fitness*, May 2009, 312.
Quick and interesting read on phytonutrients.

Tabatha, Elliot. "The Nutrition Notebook: The Buck Stops Here," *Muscle and Fitness*, May 2009, 314.
Great article on buckwheat protein.

Fish Oll

Maroon, JC and JW Bost. "Omega-3 Fatty Acids (Fish Oil) as an Anti-inflammatory: An Alternative to Nonsteroidal Anti-inflammatory Drugs for Discogenic Pain." *Surgical Neurology* 65, no. 4 (April 2006):326–331.
A very interesting study for anyone with chronic joint injuries.

Brown, Jordan. "Go Fish." *Musclemag,* June 2009:217.
The effects of fish oil on insulin resistance.

Green Tea

Duloo AG, Duret C, Rohrer D, et al. "Efficacy of a Green Tea Extract Rich in Catechin Polyphenols and Caffeine in Increasing 24-h Energy Expenditure and Fat Oxidation in Humans." *Am J Clin Nutr,* 2000 Nov;72(5):1232-4.

Nagao T, Hase T, Tokimitsu I. "A Green Tea Extract High in Catechins Reduces Body Fat and Cardiovascular Risks in Humans." *Obesity.* 2007 Jun;15(6):1473-83.
Study on the fat burning potential of green tea

Lee MS, Kim CT, Kim Y. "Green Tea (-)-Epigallocatechin-3-Gallate Reduces Body Weight with Regulation of Multiple Genes Expression in Adipose Tissue of Diet-Induced Obese Mice." *Ann Nutr Metab.* 2009;54(2):151-7.

Westerterp-Plantenga MS, Lejeune MP, Kovacs EM. "Body Weight Loss and Weight Maintenance in Relation to Habitual Caffeine Intake and Green Tea Supplementation." *Obes Res.* 2005 Jul;13(7):1195-204.

Creatine

Hopkins, WG. "Creatine and Kidney Damage? Physiology and Physical Education." *Sportscience* 2000;4(1).

Poortmans JR, Francaux M. "Long-Term Oral Creatine Supplementation Does Not Impair Renal Function in Healthy Athletes." *Medicine and Science in Sports and Exercise* 31;1999:1108-1110
There is scant evidence that creatine can cause renal failure in a healthy athlete.

Candow DG, Chilibeck PD. "Effect of Creatine Supplementation During Resistance Training on Muscle Accretion in the Elderly." *J Nutr Health Aging.* 2007 Mar-Apr;11(2):185-8.
Creatine has the potential to enforce muscle hypertrophy.

Stretching

Garnett, LR. "Stretching It to the Limit: Stretching Exercises Increase Flexibility of Joints."
Harvard Health Letter, July 1996.

Bacurau RF, Monteiro GA, Ugrinowitsch C, et al. "Acute Effect of a Ballistic and a Static Stretching Exercise Bout on Flexibility and Maximal Strength. *J Strength Cond Res.* 2009 Jan;23(1):304-8.
Stretching before exercising will weaken you.

Rubini EC, Costa AL, Gomes PS. "The Effects of Stretching on Strength Performance." *Sports Med.* 2007;37(3):213-24.
Stretching works against optimal performance when done before a weight workout.

Eggs and cholesterol

Ratliff JC, Mutungi G, Puglisi MJ, et al. "Eggs Modulate the Inflammatory Response to Carbohydrate Restricted Diets in Overweight Men" *Nutr Metab (Lond).* 2008 Feb 20;5:6.
Gives a good view on how eggs can help regulate insulin and cholesterol.

Mutungi G, Ratliff J, Puglisi M, et al. "Dietary Cholesterol from Eggs Increases Plasma HDL Cholesterol in Overweight Men Consuming a Carbohydrate-Restricted Diet". *J Nutr.* 2008 Feb;138(2):272-6.
HDL (good) cholesterol elevated through the consumption of eggs.

Low-carbohydrate diets

Ratliff J, Mutungi G, Puglisi MJ, Volek JS, Fernandez ML. "Carbohydrate Restriction (with or without Additional Dietary Cholesterol Provided by Eggs) Reduces Insulin Resistance and Plasma Leptin without Modifying Appetite Hormones in Adult Men." *Nutr Res.* 2009 Apr;29(4):262-8.

Nordmann AJ, Nordmann A, Briel M, et al. "Effects of Low-Carbohydrate vs Low-Fat Diets on Weight Loss and Cardiovascular Risk Factors: A Meta-Analysis of Randomized Controlled Trials." *Arch Intern Med.* 2006 Feb 13;166(3):285-93.
Low-carb diets without energy restrictions are as effective for weight loss as energy-restricted regular diets.

Thomas DE, Elliott EJ, Baur L. "Low Glycaemic Index or Low

Glycaemic Load Diets for Overweight and Obesity." *Cochrane Database Syst Rev.* 2007 Jul 18;(3):CD005105.
Controlling insulin might be one of the most crucial points for diet success.

Leite JO, DeOgburn R, Ratliff JC, et al. "Low-Carbohydrate Diet Disrupts the Association Between Insulin Resistance and Weight Gain. *Metabolism.* 2009 Aug;58(8):1116-22.
The association between weight gain and insulin resistance appears to be dependent on high carbohydrate intakes.

Lobley GE, Bremner DM, Holtrop G, et al. "Impact of High-Protein Diets with Either Moderate or Low Carbohydrate on Weight Loss, Body Composition, Blood Pressure and Glucose Tolerance in Rats. *Br J Nutr.* 2007 Jun;97(6):1099-108.
Lowered fasting insulin through such a diet might help with obesity-related diseases.

Fructose

Stanhope KL, Havel PJ. "Fructose Consumption: Considerations for Future Research on Its Effects on Adipose Distribution, Lipid Metabolism, and Insulin Sensitivity in Humans." *J Int Soc Sports Nutr.* 2009 Jan 28;6:4.utr. 2009 Jun;139(6):1236S-1241.
Increased consumption of fructose can lead to additional visceral adipose tissue buildup

Sweeteners

Nakagawa Y, Nagasawa M, Yamada S, et al. "Sweet Taste Receptor Expressed in Pancreatic Beta-Cells Activates the Calcium and Cyclic AMP Signaling Systems and Stimulates Insulin Secretion." *PLoS One.* 2009;4(4):e5106.
The insulin response from diet drinks is almost as high as from sugar sodas

Abou-Donia MB, El-Masry EM, Abdel-Rahman AA, et al. "Splenda Alters Gut Microflora and Increases Intestinal P-Glycoprotein and Cytochrome P-450 in Male Rats: *Journal of Toxicology and Environmental Health*, Part A, Volume 71, Issue 21 January 2008,1415–1429.
The dangers of sweeteners.

One popular fat burner study

Bloomer RJ, Fisher-Wellman KH, Hammond KG, et al. "Dietary Supplement Increases Plasma Norepinephrine, Lipolysis, and Metabolic Rate in Resistance Trained Men." *J Int Soc Sports Nutr.* 2009 Apr 17;6:10.

Topical fat loss creams

Caruso MK, Pekarovic S, Raum WJ, et al. "Topical Fat Reduction from the Waist." *Diabetes Obes Metab.* 2007 May;9(3):300-3.

Dickinson BI, Gora-Harper ML. "Aminophylline for Cellulite Removal." *Ann Pharmacother.* 1996 Mar;30(3):292-3.
The combination of yohimbine and aminophylline holds promise.

Cardio

Lunn WR, Finn JA, Axtell RS. "Effects of Sprint Interval Training and Body Weight Reduction on Power to Weight Ratio in Experienced Cyclists." *Strength Cond Res.* 2009 Jul;23(4):1217-24.

LaForgia J, Withers RT, Gore CJ. Effects of Exercise Intensity and Duration of Post-Exercise Oxygen Consumption. *J Sports Sci.* (2006) 24(12):1247-64.
Good review on why the difference between HIIT and low-intensity cardio is smaller than assumed.

Why excessive cardio will lower your BMR

Poehlman ET, Melby CL, Goran MI. "The Impact of Exercise and Diet Restriction on Daily Energy Expenditure." *Sports Med.* 1991 Feb;11(2):78-101.
Doing too much cardio will cause muscle loss, thereby lowering your BMR.

Role of strength training and extra protein in a diet as opposed to a simple low-calorie, cardio approach

Stegler P, Cunliffe A. "The Role of Diet and Exercise for the Maintenance of Fat-Free Mass and Resting Metabolic Rate during Weight Loss." *Sports Med.* 2006;36(3):239-62.
A high-protein diet with strength training is more effective than a simple calorie cutting approach

Training for older men

Craig BW, Everhart J, Brown R. "The Influence of High-Resistance Training on Glucose Tolerance in Young and Elderly Subjects." *Mech Ageing Dev.* 1989 Aug;49(2):147-57.
Resistance training improves glucose tolerance in older athletes

Nicklas BJ, Ryan AJ, Treuth MM, et al. "Testosterone, Growth Hormone and IGF-I Responses to Acute and Chronic Resistive Exercise in Men Aged 55-70 Years." *Int J Sports Med.* 1995 Oct;16(7):445-50.
Study shows that weight training can have a positive effect on hormones in older men.

Red wine

Sato M, Maulik N, Das DK. "Cardioprotection with Alcohol: Role of both Alcohol and Polyphenolic Antioxidants." *Ann N Y Acad Sci.* 2002 May;957:122-35.
Both alcohol and anti-oxidants from red wine play a role in heart health

Spinach

Rutzke CJ, Glahn RP, Rutzke MA, et al. "Bioavailability of Iron from Spinach Using an In Vitro/Human Caco-2 Cell Bioassay Model." *Habitation (Elmsford).* 2004;10(1):7-14.
Spinach is actually a poor source of iron.

Overeating

Oakes ME. "Filling Yet Fattening: Stereotypical Beliefs about the Weight Gain Potential and Satiation of Foods." *Appetite.* 2006 Mar;46(2):224-33.
Shows how dieters are wrong about their caloric intake estimates.

Refeeds/cheat day

Bigrigg JK, Heigenhauser GJ, Inglis JG, et al. "Carbohydrate Re-Feeding after a High-Fat Diet Rapidly Reverses the Adaptive Increase in Human Skeletal Muscle PDH Kinase Activity." *Am J Physiol Regul Integr Comp Physiol.* 2009 Jul 22.
A higher carb day can offset muscle loss incurred from a diet.

Paleo Diet

Cordain L, Eaton SB, Sebastian A, et al. "Origins and Evolution of the Western Diet: Health Implications for the 21st Century." Am J Clin Nutr. 2005 Feb;81(2):341-54.
Looks at newer (in terms of human consumption) foods, such as grains and sugar, and their implications for our health.

High-intensity cardio versus low-intensity cardio with regard to fat loss

van Aggel-Leijssen DP, Saris WH, Wagenmakers AJ, et al. "Effect of Exercise Training at Different Intensities on Fat Metabolism of Obese Men." J Appl Physiol. 2002 Mar;92(3):1300-9.
In untrained people and beginners, there is little need to perform HIIT.

Utilization of nutrients during exercise

Kanaley JA, Weatherup-Dentes MM, Alvarado CR, et al. "Substrate Oxidation during Acute Exercise and with Exercise Training in Lean and Obese Women. *Eur J Appl Physiol.* 2001 Jul;85(1-2):68-73.
Athletes utilize very little fat during exercise, hence diet plays an even greater role.

Weight lifting benefits for women

Parker-Pope, T. "Weight Lifting May Help to Avert Lymph Problem" *The New York Times.* August 18, 2009.

Protein and fat loss

Noakes M. "The Role of Protein in Weight Management." *Asia Pac J Clin Nutr.* 2008;17 Suppl 1:169-71.
Protein speeds weight loss through its ability to increase satiety.
Brehm BJ, D'Alessio DA. "Benefits of High-Protein Weight Loss Diets: Enough Evidence for Practice?" *Curr Opin Endocrinol Diabetes Obes.* 2008 Oct;15(5):416-21.

Halton TL, Hu FB. "The Effects of High Protein Diets on Thermogenesis, Satiety and Weight Loss: a Critical Review." *J Am Coll Nutr.* 2004 Oct;23(5):373-85.
Both studies show that a high-protein diet has a higher success rate than carb-based diets

Weight training and fat loss

Kerksick CM, Wilborn CD, Campbell BI, et al. "Early-Phase Adaptations to a Split-Body, Linear Periodization Resistance Traning Program in College-Aged and Middle-Aged Men." *J Strength Cond Res.* 2009 May;23(3):962-71.Click here to read Links
Study shows how effective weight training is for fat loss.

Post workout shake

Chromiak JA, Smedley B, Carpenter W, et al. "Effect of a 10-Week Strength Training Program and Recovery Drink on Body Composition, Muscular Strength and Endurance, and Anaerobic Power and Capacity." *Nutrition.* 2004 May;20(5):420-7.
Provides some evidence that a post workout shake will help gain fat free mass (FFM) faster.

Sport drinks

Almiron-Roig E, Drewnowski A. "Hunger, Thirst, and Energy Intakes Following Consumption of Caloric Beverages." *Physiol Behav.* 2003 Sep;79(4-5):767-73.
Soft drinks do not subdue hunger effectively, despite their caloric content.

Varanian LR, Schwartz MB, Brownell KD. "Effects of Soft Drink Consumption on Nutrition and Health: A Systematic Review and

Meta-Analysis." *Am J Public Health*. 2007 Apr;97(4):667-75.
Overconsumption of sport and soft drinks leads to health issues.

Soy and testosterone

Hamilton-Reeves JM, Vazquez G, Duval SJ, et al. "Clinical Studies Show No Effects of Soy Protein or Isoflavones on Reproductive Hormones in Men: Results of a Meta-Analysis." *Fertil Steril*. 2009 Jun 11.
Comprehensive study showing that soy does not have any measurable effect on testosterone.

Zhuo XG, Melby MK, Watanabe S. "Soy Isoflavone Intake Lowers Serum LDL Cholesterol: A Meta-Analysis of 8 Randomized Controlled Trials in Humans." *J Nutr*. 2004 Sep;134(9):2395-400.
Cholesterol-lowering properties of soy protein.

BCAAs
Blomstrand E, Eliasson J, Karlsson HK, et al. "Branched-Chain Amino Acids Activate Key Enzymes in Protein Synthesis after Physical Exercise. *J Nutr*. 2006 Jan;136(1 Suppl):269S-73S.
BCAAs can be helpful in suppressing catabolism during the workout.

Whey

Hayes A, Cribb PJ. "Effect of Whey Protein Isolate on Strength, Body Composition and Muscle Hypertrophy during Resistance Training." *Curr Opin Clin Nutr Metab Care*. 2008 Jan;11(1):40-4.
The favorable effect of whey protein on body composition

Steroids

Hartgens F, Kuipers H. "Effects of Androgenic-Anabolic Steroids in Athletes." *Sports Med*. 2004;34(8):513-54.
The good, the bad, the ugly on steroids

Simon P, Striegel H, Aust F, et al. "Doping in Fitness Sports: Estimated Number of Unreported Cases and Individual Probability of Doping." *Addiction* 2006 Nov;101(11):1640-4.

Between 15 and 20% of all gym goers are said to have used steroids at one point in their training.

Training for kids and young adults

McGuigan MR, Tatasciore M, Newton RU, et al. "Eight Weeks of Resistance Training Can Significantly Alter Body Composition in Children Who Are Overweight or Obese."
J Strength Cond Res. 2009 Jan;23(1):80-5.

Castro MJ, McCann DJ, Shaffrath JD, et al. "Peak Torque per Unit Cross-Sectional Area Differs Between Strength-Trained and Untrained Young Adults." *Med Sci Sports Exerc. 1996 Jul;28(7):934-5.*
How young adults and children can benefit from weight training.

Hardgainer

Orvanová E. "Somatotypes of Weight Lifters." *J Sports Sci.* 1990 Summer;8(2):119-37.
A brief study of somatypes found in different weight classes in wrestling.

HIT

Rønnestad BR, Egeland W, Kvamme NH, et al. "Dissimilar Effects of One- and Three-Set Strength Training on Strength and Muscle Mass Gains in Upper and Lower Body in Untrained Subjects." *J Strength Cond Res.* 2007 Feb;21(1):157-63.
Shows that three sets per exercise are more efficient than just one.

Paulsen G, Myklestad D, Raastad T. "The Influence of Volume of Exercise on Early Adaptations to Strength Training." *J Strength Conditioning Res.* 2003 Feb;17(1):115-20.
Another study that shows the necessity of multiple sets.

Baar K, Esser K. "Phosphorylation of p70(S6k) Correlates with Increased Skeletal Muscle Mass Following Resistance Exercise." *Am J Physiol.* 1999 Jan;276(1 Pt 1):C120-7.

www.ingramcontent.com/pod-product-compliance
Lightning Source LLC
Chambersburg PA
CBHW06 303280526
45784CB00002B/880